BREAST CANCER HUSBAND

HOW TO HELP YOUR WIFE (AND YOURSELF) THROUGH DIAGNOSIS, TREATMENT, AND BEYOND

MARC SILVER

Foreword by medical oncologist Frederick P. Smith, M.D.

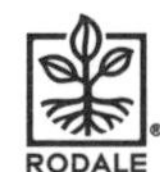

Notice

This book is intended as a reference volume only, not as a medical manual. The information given here is designed to help you make informed decisions about your health. It is not intended as a substitute for any treatment that may have been prescribed by your doctor. If you suspect that you have a medical problem, we urge you to seek competent medical help.

Mention of specific companies, organizations, or authorities in this book does not imply endorsement by the author or publisher, nor does mention of specific companies, organizations, or authorities imply that they endorse this book, its author, or the publisher.

Internet addresses and telephone numbers given in this book were accurate at the time it went to press.

Printed in the United States of America

Rodale Inc. makes every effort to use acid-free ♾, recycled paper ♻.

Michael Kelly's quotation on page 75 is reprinted with permission from *The Washington Post* Writers Group © 2001.
"Sizing Up a Tumor" on page 117 is reprinted from the 2003 Mammography Card with the permission of the Susan G. Komen Breast Cancer Foundation.
The information on cancer stages that appears on pages 118-119 is adapted with permission from www.breastcancer.org, a nonprofit organization that provides in-depth information about breast cancer.
Information used for the Glossary on pages 295-300 is reprinted with permission from the American Cancer Society's "Breast Cancer Dictionary" and from www.breastcancer.org's "Talking Dictionary."

Book design by UDG/DesignWorks

Library of Congress Cataloging-in-Publication Data

Silver, Marc, date.
Breast cancer husband : how to help your wife (and yourself) through diagnosis, treatment, and beyond / Marc Silver ; foreword by Frederick P. Smith.
p. cm.
Includes index.
ISBN 1–57954–833–4 paperback
1. Breast—Cancer—Popular works. 2. Breast—Cancer—Patients—Family relationships. 3. Breast—Cancer—Psychological aspects. 4. Husbands. 5. Caregivers. I. Title.
RC280.B8S4972 2004
616.99'449—dc22 2004007914

Distributed to the trade by Holtzbrinck Publishers

4 6 8 10 9 7 5 3 paperback

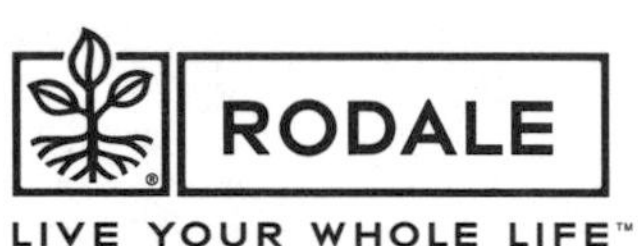

Advance praise for *Breast Cancer Husband*

"No one should face breast cancer alone. But how does a husband support his wife when he may be feeling frustrated, sad, and angry himself? Author Marc Silver fills an essential niche with his book, Breast Cancer Husband, *offering emotional support and practical advice to help men be compassionate caregivers—everything from tips for talking to children to a frank discussion of sexuality and intimacy."*

—Nancy G. Brinker,
founder of the Susan G. Komen Breast Cancer Foundation

"When cancer happens, it happens to the entire family—not just the person with the diagnosis. Marc Silver knows this and—thank goodness—has written an honest, informative and, yes, even humorous guide for breast cancer husbands. A must-read for every man who's learning to live with breast cancer."

—Diane Perlmutter, CEO, Gilda's Club Worldwide

"A clear, concise crash-course that lists the best ways to help when a man sets out to support his wife through the ordeal of breast cancer."

—William H. Goodson, III, M.D.
breast surgeon and clinical research scientist, San Francisco

"Breast Cancer Husband *bravely and honestly discusses topics—including talking with your children about the diagnosis, the nuances of diagnosis and therapy, and intimacy issues—that men need to understand to be helpful, supportive partners in the battle against cancer."*

—Mikkael Sekeres, M.D., staff oncologist,
at the Cleveland Clinic Foundation and author of *Facing Cancer*

"If the woman in your life has breast cancer, you will likely feel less alone, and more confident in your skills to support her emotionally and practically, after reading this book. Marc Silver deftly blends expert advice, personal accounts, and the latest research to create a lively and highly readable resource for men who love a breast cancer survivor."

—Leslie R. Schover, Ph.D., professor of behavioral science,
University of Texas M.D. Anderson Cancer Center

"Marc Silver has written the book that every woman faced with a diagnosis of breast cancer will want her husband to read. It's honest, engaging, and inspirational. I will highly recommend it to congregants and clients."

—The Reverend Debra W. Haffner
director, Religious Institute on Sexual Morality, Justice, and Healing

"The only book of its kind, Breast Cancer Husband *offers straightforward, honest, easy-to-read information that will help husbands and their spouses deal with this devastating disease. If only we had had Marc Silver as our mentor when we got the diagnosis of breast cancer with its maze of decisions and emotions! His book is truly a Godsend."*

—Allen and Linda Anderson, coauthors of *Angel Cats: Divine Messengers of Comfort* and founders of the Angel Animals Network

"Indisputably, the crushing burden of breast cancer falls on the woman. Yet husbands soon learn that they too have plenty of picking up to do: the slack, her spirits, the house, the pieces. Marc Silver's book helps husbands cope."

—Jack Burlingame, breast cancer husband and founding board member of the breast cancer group Men With Heart (menwithheart.org)

"I read this book through in a single sitting, and I was immediately struck by the commonality of experience among all of us breast cancer husbands. As different and varied as our stories may be, we all share many consistent elements. That, I think, is what makes this book invaluable to any man who is faced with being a breast cancer husband. The knowledge that many other men have felt the same fear, uncertainty, sadness, and guilt when confronting this disease in their closest loved one cannot be overvalued. Example: Who knew there were other "car criers?" All this time I thought it was just me! There is no sugarcoating in this book: it is a sometimes brutally realistic look at the reality of living with cancer, with just enough science to make it informative and a liberal dose of gentle but very necessary humor. A must-have for any (reluctant) breast cancer husband. I only wish I had the benefit of this book during my rude introduction to the world of breast cancer."

—Frank Sadowski, vice president, Consumer Electronics Merchandising, amazon.com, and breast cancer husband

To the women who have taught me how to be a better man:
my mother, Shirley,
my daughters, Maya and Daniela,
and, especially, my wife, Marsha

Contents

Foreword

Does the world need yet another book on breast cancer?

Bookstores and libraries carry dozens of books about this disease. Many of these breast cancer books do an excellent job explaining the nature of the disease. From my work as a medical oncologist who treats many breast cancer patients—and from my own experience as the husband of a breast cancer survivor—I know only too well how devastating it is when cancer is diagnosed, and how overwhelming the consequences of that discovery can be. A well-researched text can add a new perspective to consider, a clarification, a way of deciding which of the many avenues of treatment to pursue.

But there is a significant gap in the literature of breast cancer. Of the 210,000 women in the United States who are diagnosed each year, many go through treatment with their husband by their side. Yet books that speak directly to the husband are rare.

Breast Cancer Husband is true to its title: This book was written by a journalist whose wife was diagnosed with this malignancy. It is one of the few breast cancer books to speak directly to the husband as he partners with his wife on this unwelcome journey.

Written from the husband's perspective, the book seeks to provide the spouse with the information he needs to comprehend what his wife is going through—and to help her as she ponders the necessary treatment decisions that she must make in this most turbulent of times in a family's life. Drawing upon his abilities as a reporter, the author has interviewed surgeons and oncologists who treat breast cancer patients, as well as the women (and their husbands) who have learned by going through treatment themselves. Using their information and insights as well as his own experience, he navigates the maze of treatment options, the vagaries of each treatment, the frustration of not knowing the answers to so many questions: Why did this happen? What can we do to prevent it from happening again? What does the future hold?

This book plays another vital role as well. The husband of a breast cancer patient is a bystander. But he, too, is traumatized by the diagnosis, and is desperate to lighten in any way possible the burden his wife must bear. Yet as the husband goes to doctor's appointments with his wife, the doctor typically does not have time to counsel him on his role. In this book, you will find answers to many of the questions you will face, from the mundane matter of what to prepare for dinner after a chemotherapy session to the awkward question of how to maintain a sense of intimacy in a relationship when your wife is reeling from the detection of a potentially lethal condition.

Breast Cancer Husband will be helpful to husbands in many ways, and perhaps in no more important way than to reinforce the lesson that I have learned as I have seen couples go through treatment together: the support of a spouse can make a significant difference to the patient. At a time when a woman's world is bowled over, when her optimism and confidence in the future is greatly tested and she is suffering the sudden loss of blissful ignorance, her husband can be a source of emotional strength, providing a shoulder to lean on. The patient has an ally when going to the doctor's office, where the information she receives may be unpleasant or frightening, regardless of how it is provided. If a patient comes alone, she may be completely mixed up by the information she hears. She has no foil to echo what happened in the office. The comfort of having a husband—one willing to subjugate his needs and schedule and time to help her—has to be of immeasurable benefit.

Yet it is deceptively hard to give the kind of support a patient needs. The husband has to understand that he is not the patient. His wife is. The breast cancer husband will at times be frustrated and overwhelmed. But as you will see when you read this book, such emotions are perfectly normal. And readers of this book will gain insights into how a husband might cope with such feelings as he seeks to provide solace and support for his wife.

So is this just another book on breast cancer? The answer is a resounding NO! The unique perspective it provides is a welcome addition to the breast cancer bookshelf.

Frederick P. Smith, M.D.,
medical oncologist affiliated with Sibley Memorial Hospital in Washington, D.C.

Acknowledgments

I must first thank the excellent doctors who cared for my wife, Marsha, and who shared their knowledge with me as I researched this book: breast surgeon Cynthia Drogula, M.D., medical oncologist Fred Smith, M.D., and radiation oncologist Irene Gage, M.D. Their expertise was invaluable.

I knew there was a book to be done after I spent an afternoon with Lillie Shockney, breast cancer survivor and director of education and outreach at the Johns Hopkins Breast Center in Baltimore. She regaled me with funny and poignant stories from her own experience as well as from her work with patients and the men she calls their "significant sweeties." I am deeply indebted to Lillie for reading the manuscript and patiently correcting my medical miscues. For any breast cancer husband looking for a gift for his wife, I highly recommend her hilarious and helpful memoir, *Breast Cancer Survivors' Club: A Nurse's Experience.*

Breast surgeon Theodore Tsangaris, M.D., medical director of the Johns Hopkins Breast Center, gave me the opportunity to gain the doctor's perspective on breast cancer when he invited me to observe a lumpectomy and a mastectomy. After I saw how much poking and prodding goes on in a lumpectomy, I went home and gave my wife an extra big hug.

Philadelphia breast radiation oncologist Marisa Weiss, M.D., brilliantly deconstructed the husband's role at a doctor's appointment—and always had time for one more question on topics from tumor size to sex toys.

I am grateful to all the breast cancer experts who spent time with me in person and on the phone, and who reviewed chapters as well—with special thanks to oncologist Sharon Giordano, M.D., of the M.D. Anderson Cancer Center in Houston, for always finding time for one more chapter, and to Richard Ogden, Ph.D., the psychologist who leads the breast cancer husband support group that I attend, for his thoughtful critique. My fellow support group members, Jim, David, and Paul, kept me on the right track with their honest accounts of their feelings and fears. My dear friend Deborah Zarin, M.D., always had time to field a medical query from out of the blue.

My researcher, David Grimm, was a first-rate interviewer and information gatherer in the final crunch. My good colleagues (and good friends) Katy Kelly and Linda Kulman offered critiques that were important in shaping this book. James Bock's keen editing eye thoroughly improved the manuscript. I couldn't have written this book without the News You Can Use wisdom I learned from Avery Comarow. And I deeply appreciate the support of my boss, Brian Duffy, and of all my colleagues at *U.S. News & World Report*.

Susan Shinagawa, past chair of the Intercultural Cancer Council and herself a breast cancer survivor, connected me with some extraordinary breast cancer husbands. So did the Susan G. Komen Breast Cancer Foundation, Gilda's Club, www.breastcancer.org, Y-ME National Breast Cancer Organization, Men Against Breast Cancer, and Men with Heart, a great group of guys who participate in breast cancer walkathons in the Boston area. I couldn't have met the pledge requirements for the Avon walk without their generous assistance. And I am especially grateful for the hospitality of my Bostonian sister-in-law, Arlene Dale.

My indefatigable agent, Stephanie Kip Rostan, believed in this project from the start. Without her commitment, there would be no book. And I can't even begin to express my gratitude to my wonderful editor, Deanna Portz, who helped persuade Rodale to publish this title. I also thank Lois Hazel for her attention to so many details as the book's project manager.

Above all, this book owes its existence to the many husbands who told me their stories with honesty, heartfelt emotion, and good humor. I feel as close to these men as to any friend I've ever had. We've all been in the trenches together.

Even if I could say thank you in every language on earth, I'd still need to find more ways to express my appreciation to my wife, Marsha. She put up with my questions at a time when she really didn't want to be thinking about cancer every single day, read chapters and offered her insights, and tolerated my absentee husbandism while I was hunched over the laptop. Marsha, you are my lover, my friend, my confidante, and my inspiration.

Introduction

In September 2001, I became a member of a club I really didn't want to join. My wife, Marsha Dale, was diagnosed with breast cancer, and I became a breast cancer husband.

As we stumbled from doctor to doctor, fought with our HMO to obtain the appropriate care, and wondered what to do about the disease that had invaded our lives, I kept wishing I had a manual to guide me. True, men aren't the lead actors in this drama, but a spouse or boyfriend can play a vital supporting role. And it sure would be nice to have a collection of cue cards for those inevitable awkward moments, both in the doctor's office and on the home front.

I wanted to know what I was supposed to do at doctor's appointments, especially when a physician seemed to be pushing my wife in directions that weren't comfortable for her. I wanted to know how to comfort my wife when her face looked more sorrowful than I'd ever seen. And I wanted to know what to do about the span of emotions I was feeling—sometimes in tune with Marsha, and sometimes at the opposite end of the spectrum.

Above all, I was petrified that I'd say or do the wrong thing. If you goof up on Valentine's Day or forget your wife's birthday, you can always make amends next year. But when your wife is fighting a life-threatening disease, you want to be on top of your game. The problem is, you've never been on the playing field before. Of course, you're not alone in your ineptitude. Most guys are complete novices when it comes to this caregiving thing.

Part of this book is a medical guide—a crash course for husbands so they will know what to expect and what questions they can help their wives ask. Breast cancer is a highly individualized disease, and the patient herself must make many decisions along the way, guided by her medical team and her own instincts. As she tries to figure out what to do, she may need the help of her spouse. Sometimes the husband hears the doctor's words more clearly than his wife, who may be too shocked and anguished to take it all in.

Many other books and Web sites cover the medical side of breast cancer. My ultimate goal is to give husbands a better understanding of how to support and care for their wives during the months of treatment and beyond—everything from what to say to a bald wife to what to do about intimacy (or the lack of it).

I spoke to dozens of social workers, psychologists, and psychiatrists who shared their insights into the impact cancer has on a marriage, and who told me much I wish I had known as Marsha went through her months of treatment.

But the people who taught me the most were breast cancer couples—the women and men who together fight the disease. I interviewed nearly 100 veterans of the breast cancer wars. They showed me that there is no one way to be a breast cancer husband. Really, it's whatever *she* wants you to be.

And I've learned that the most important task for a breast cancer husband is to be there for his wife, and to listen to what she's saying. I know, I know—it sounds so vague and feel-goodish, but that's the essence of your job.

Those men and women who talked to me with candor and humor and sometimes tears—they are the heart and soul of this book. They made me laugh with outrageous tales of wigs gone astray, and they made me cry as they shared their innermost thoughts and fears. In a few cases, because of the sensitive nature of their comments, the interviewees asked to be identified by a pseudonym. Those names are marked with an asterisk. But most of them agreed to let me use their names along with their remarks.

With breast cancer, there is always a fear of recurrence. I interviewed a number of couples who are living with metastatic disease—breast cancer that has spread to the bones or other organs in the body. Their courage is extraordinary; several chapters in this book tell how these brave women (and their husbands) live with hope—and, in some cases, face death with incredible bravery. Three of the women I interviewed died from the disease a few months after we spoke—a tragic reminder that, despite the great progress in treatment, sometimes there is nothing doctors can do. I am grateful to have had the chance to speak with these three courageous souls: Trish Como, Brenda Heil, and Carol Shields.

My fervent hope for all my readers—the brotherhood of breast cancer husbands—is that your wife will fare well. That one day soon, your biggest problem will be figuring out what to tell well-meaning acquaintances who say, "They got all the cancer, and your wife is going to be fine, right?" And that you will be able to reply, as I do, "Well, they never know for sure with breast cancer, but I can tell you this: Marsha is feeling good."

Part I

Dealing with the Diagnosis

Unwelcome to the World of Breast Cancer

What to do in those frantic early days

When the news came, I was a husband behaving badly.

It was the last Friday of August 2001. The phone in my office rang around 11:00 A.M. My wife's voice, shrouded by cell-phone static, sounded raw and uneasy. I knew she had gone to the doctor for a follow-up mammogram. A reading earlier that week had raised eyebrows. But Marsha, who was 53, had had plenty of callbacks before, and neither of us was particularly nervous about this one. She thought it was a nuisance that she had to run back to the HMO for what undoubtedly would prove to be a false alarm. Needless to say, I didn't bother to go along.

So my wife went in, unsnapped her bra, and placed her naked right breast in the grip of the mammogram machine. The technician gave the image to the radiologist to examine. A few minutes later, the doctor came into the room where Marsha was putting on her clothes, and with six little words catapulted her into the world of breast cancer: "Sure looks like cancer to me."

Deeply distraught, Marsha called me as soon as she was out of the doctor's office. She wanted to share her pain and to seek some husbandly solace. On a scale of 1 to 10, with 10 being truly superb and 1 being utterly inadequate, my reaction deserved, oh, maybe a minus 11. And I'm being a lenient grader. My wife still likes to remind me of my exact (and insipid) words: "Ew, that doesn't sound good."

We spoke for only a few minutes on that balmy summer Friday as we headed into Labor Day weekend—mainly about logistics (because they're a heck of a lot easier to talk about than feelings). Marsha couldn't see a surgeon until Tuesday because of the holiday. Nothing we could do about that. We decided we wouldn't say anything to our two daughters (they were 12 and 15 at the time) until we knew for sure . . . because the doctor could be wrong, right? And then I said something like, "I'll be home at the usual time." What was I thinking? Yes, what was I thinking?

I'm sure that question must have crossed my wife's mind.

"Women always ask what men are thinking about," comedian Jerry Seinfeld says in one of his monologues. "We're thinking about nothing. We're just walking down the street, not thinking about anything." I believe that was my goal at the time. I didn't want to think about anything.

But, truth be told, my mind was working overtime. Deep inside, I was shocked and scared. I may have been 49, but I felt as if I were 14. I didn't know how we'd muddle through the next 3 anxious days until we saw the surgeon. And if the radiologist proved to be correct, I couldn't even begin to imagine how we'd cope in the months ahead.

YOUR FIRST REACTION

Of all the words in the medical lexicon, "cancer" is the most terrifying, says Jim Zabora, Sc.D., a social worker who has counseled cancer patients for years and is now dean of the Catholic University of America's School of Social Service in Washington, D.C. Breast cancer husbands agree 100 percent.

"You are absolutely shattered," recalls Stephen Peck of Washington, D.C., whose wife, Gayle, was diagnosed when she was 41. "You can't believe it. Why did she get it? She had no family history, no nothing." A ruddy fellow who'd look at home on a golf course, Stephen recalls, "I absolutely bawled my eyes out. You are in total shock and fear because you don't know what's going to happen."

"It was just like somebody punched me in the gut," says Chicagoan Bob Marovich, 39, who felt the lump in his wife's breast before she was aware of it, kept the secret over a holiday weekend, then told her. After having a biopsy, she went for a follow-up visit to the doctor and got the news that the lump was malignant. That's when she called Bob at the office. "I remember not hearing anything else people had to say at work after I heard the news. I went home, and even though you don't want to jump to conclusions, your emotions do."

There's a term for the swirl of emotions you feel in the days after a cancer diagnosis: "acute stress reaction." The symptoms are "shock, disbelief, and

---

THE KINDNESS OF STRANGERS

In the middle of the hectic early days of breast cancer, we somehow missed sending off a credit card payment on time. Sure enough, we got socked with a penalty the next month.

So I called the credit card company and told them the truth: "My wife was just diagnosed with breast cancer, and some of the bills in the house didn't get prompt attention."

The penalty was erased. And a little lightbulb went on. I realized that although breast cancer was playing havoc with our sense of stability and immortality, it had given us something, too. We had the perfect excuse for all our screwups. So we took advantage. I mean, why not? It wasn't as if we were lying.

"I do tell people, the cancer is taking enough away from you—use it to gain stuff," advises Frank McCaffrey, a clinical social worker who counsels breast cancer husbands at Boston's Beth Israel Deaconess Medical Center. "Maybe your wife is more likely to get seated at a restaurant when she wears a scarf. If it's going to get you a little something extra, why not? Drop it into conversation. People will feel bad and want to make it up to you. And that's okay."

Marsha and I discovered that a mere mention of the disease is a highly effective way to get an annoying telephone solicitor off the line. It's a powerful weapon when you're fighting, um, negotiating with your health insurer. And when a gift card expires because you couldn't get to the store in the middle of the chemo months, there's nothing wrong with seeing if the manager will show a little breast cancer sympathy.

numbness," says Margie Stohner, a licensed clinical social worker and consultant to the psychosocial program at Sibley Memorial Hospital's Center for Breast Health in Washington, D.C.

Though the woman is the one who has the disease, the man in her life is inextricably bound up in the emotions of the moment. "I think it's tough to be the husband," says Cynthia Drogula, M.D., who is a breast surgeon in Washington, D.C. Breast cancer patients agree. "Women say, 'I think it's harder on my poor husband,'" says Judy Perotti, former director of patient services for Y-ME National Breast Cancer Organization, which runs a support hotline for patients and their spouses.

Understandably, nobody asks the husband how he's feeling. All the attention is on the wife, and the husband is just expected to be there for her in some vague, undefined way. The same applies to boyfriends, significant others, fiancés, and long-term companions, all of whom I think of as honorary breast cancer husbands. Guys, this book is for you, too. (Although to keep things simple, I'll be using the terms "husband" and "wife.")

Some men, like me, don't exactly rise to the occasion when the call comes. Like the fellow who said to his newlywed wife, "I thought you were healthy when I married you." Or the husband whose first question to the doctor was, "What do I tell my friends?" Or the man who sat in the doctor's office with a poker face and his arms folded across his chest, clearly signaling that he couldn't wait to get the hell out of there.

Even with the best of intentions, you might make a fool of yourself. Riding home on the bus with his girlfriend not 30 minutes after the doctor gave her the news, Mike Malone was trying to think of a way to take her mind off breast cancer. Mike knew she was interested in buying a car, so he blurted out, "Want to go car shopping?"

The second he said it, he knew it was just about the stupidest thing he'd ever said. "If there's only one time you forget something I said," he told Stacy, "please forget that." In the 3 years since, she's never brought it up. Mike, now 35, gave her the engagement ring sooner than he'd planned. His message to breast cancer husbands: "No matter what, you're going to screw up."

But at least Mike was by Stacy's side. A woman in her 70s once came into the Johns Hopkins Breast Center in Baltimore all alone, to discuss what

GUY TALK

> **"We were raised to take things as they come. We didn't sit and moan and look for excuses and say 'Why me?' When Connie was diagnosed, we just said, 'What are the options?'"**
>
> **—RAY ELLINGER, 66**
> **Grand Rapids, Michigan**

to do about the cancerous tumor in her breast. "Do you have a significant sweetie?" asked Lillie Shockney, the warmhearted nurse who serves as director of education and outreach at the center, and who is a breast cancer survivor. "No, honey, but I've got a husband," the patient told Shockney. "But he ain't no good."

Or maybe he just didn't know what to do. Although no one has surveyed the hundreds of thousands of husbands whose wives have suffered from breast cancer, I believe that most of us want to be loyal, brave, and loving. We want to be prepared. That's easy when you're a Boy Scout, hard when you're a breast cancer husband. Men are taught to stand alone, to be tough, and to hold in their tears—three traits that don't necessarily add up to a sterling spouse in times of crisis.

MODEL HUSBANDS

If you're looking for a role model, I did come across a few. Some guys just seem to have great reflexes, even when confronted with the news of breast cancer.

Jeffrey Berger recalls the day when he got the same kind of call I did. His wife, Diane, had felt a pea-size lump on her breastbone. Her surgeon did a needle biopsy, and the lump turned out to be malignant. Jeffrey was in his law office when Diane phoned from her doctor's exam room and said, "I think I have cancer."

"Just like that," says Jeffrey, 56. Eight years later, relaxing at his Chevy Chase, Maryland, home on a hot summer Sunday, Jeffrey is still chilled by the memory. "And I said, 'You what? You have cancer?'"

Diane said, "Yes. I'm at the doctor's office and he just got back the results."

Jeffrey said, "I'll come right over." And he did. Jeffrey's father was a policeman, his uncle was a fire chief, and he was raised to follow in their footsteps: Always be ready to deal with an emergency. He knew he had to get to the doctor's office and find out what was going on.

Then comes the hard part: figuring out what to say. You couldn't do better than to take a lesson from Al Shockney, husband of Johns Hopkins nurse Lillie. He walked into his home after a late-night job driving a limo round-trip from Baltimore to New York City. A few days earlier, Lillie had had a biopsy for what appeared to be a cyst. Al, who's got a tattoo on his forearm, a neat white beard, and a twinkle in his eye, was sure everything would be fine. But then, on the long drive home, he began to wonder how he would react if it wasn't. "I knew no matter what the news was I wasn't going to sit down in a chair and break out in a cold sweat," he says. "I didn't want Lillie to see that. I was going to play it real cool. I was going to tell her whatever I could to try to relieve her mind."

Lillie, meanwhile, didn't know what she would say. She practiced in front of the mirror, trying to find the right words to tell her husband that the lump was malignant. And then when Al walked in the door, Lillie blurted out, "I have breast cancer."

Al was very calm, Lillie remembers, and asked, "Are you sure?" She was, since she had seen the biopsy report with her own eyes. Al is one of those rare men who knows just what his wife needs to hear. "I have known you a long time," Al said. "I know you are strong, with a zest for living, and we are going to be here for each other; we are going to be fine." Lillie's puckish eyes still tear up, 10 years after this conversation. "It was very convincing," she says.

At the time, Lillie didn't know what was really going on in Al's mind: "I was scared to death when she told me. My life flashed before my eyes, and everything was going by so fast. I actually wanted to cry."

Sitting in her cozy living room, Lillie laughs. "That would have been really bad for me if you did—really bad!"

BIOPSY TIME

Whether your wife's lump was found through a mammogram, a self-exam, or a doctor's exam, she will need a biopsy to learn if the lesion is benign or malignant. In Marsha's case, the doctor performed a surgical (or excisional) biopsy.

This outpatient surgery takes about an hour, but there's inevitable waiting time built in. The woman enters a twilight sleep with anesthesia delivered by IV. The surgeon cuts out all or part of the lesion, which a pathologist assesses for cancerous cells. After some of the grogginess wears off, the patient is released. She'll miss a day of work if she has a job. Biopsy results are available after several days. If the lump is malignant, the patient will then face a second surgery to remove the tumor with clear margins—that is, leaving no cancer behind.

At the time, Marsha and I didn't know there are other types of biopsies that are a lot easier on the patient: fine needle and core needle. In both cases, the needle removes a sampling of cells. The needle is a little smaller with the fine needle biopsy, which dislodges cells for examination. Cecilia Brennecke, M.D., director of breast imaging at the Johns Hopkins Breast Center at Greenspring Station in Baltimore, prefers the core biopsy, which employs a slightly larger needle. Guided by ultrasound or x-rays, the doctor removes a core of tissue from the tumor. In Dr. Brennecke's view, the result is "a much more accurate sampling" than with a fine needle.

In a needle biopsy, a local anesthetic is used. The biopsy takes about 30 minutes to an hour. Husbands sometimes come along, but Dr. Brennecke suggests they stay in the waiting room. "I think it's difficult to look at a needle biopsy," she explains, remembering one husband who fainted.

A pathologist will test the tissue for cancer. (You might want to ask how often the pathologist works with breast tumors. Weekly is an acceptable answer. Daily is even better.) Results typically come back in 1 to 3 days. Voilà: biopsy results without undergoing a surgery.

While the surgical biopsy was the "gold standard" for many years, Dr. Brennecke says, nowadays a needle biopsy should be the standard of care—the level of care a patient should expect. A study by a radiologist has found that both types of biopsies have a 98 percent accuracy rate. And with a needle biopsy, the patient does not face the risks presented by anesthesia in a surgical biopsy. In addition, there is no scarring. Keep in mind that the location or nature of the lesion could call for a surgical biopsy.

You should also realize that no biopsy is 100 percent accurate. A doctor could miss the cancerous cells in a needle sampling. And a surgeon will sometimes miss the tumor altogether in a biopsy.

That's why you want a doctor who has ample experience with breast cancer. Regardless of the type of biopsy, the results should match the doctor's initial impressions of the lesion. If the doctor deemed the lump suspicious and a needle biopsy found no cancerous cells, the doctor should investigate further. In such an instance, Cynthia Drogula, M.D., a breast surgeon who practices in Washington, D.C., might tell a patient, "This lesion has to come out anyway."

Marsha and I wonder why her docs didn't mention the option of the less invasive needle biopsy. I tried to get an answer from our HMO but no one returned my calls. The likely explanation: some doctors or health-care facilities may not have the expertise or equipment to use the needle instead of the scalpel. A needle biopsy wouldn't have changed the news about cancer. But Marsha, who, as it turned out, had a tumor in each breast, would have had two fewer surgeries to recover from.

BREAKING THE NEWS

Your wife's doctor may call and ask her to come in to his office for the results. That's pretty much the same as saying she has cancer. Dr. Brennecke favors a more direct approach: "Yes, I do tell women over the phone." If the doctor calls and suggests to your wife that she come in for the results, and she doesn't want to wait one more minute, she should definitely go ahead and ask. And she might want to have you on the other line. "I think that's good," Dr. Brennecke says. Because once the doctor utters the words, "I'm afraid it's cancer," the woman might not hear anything else. The husband is often the one who asks the question, "What do we do now?"

First, You Cry is how journalist Betty Rollin titled her breast cancer book back in 1976. That still holds true today. Next, you find a surgeon. And you'll probably find statistics for 5-year survival rates of newly diagnosed patients. They go something like this: For women diagnosed with cancer just in the breast, 97 out of 100 will be alive after 5 years; for women whose cancer has spread to the lymph nodes, 79 out of 100; and for women whose cancer has spread to her organs, 23 out of 100. "It is critically important not to hang your hat on stats," cautions Lillie Shockney. "There are people who fall on both sides of the survival curve—that's the reality." The 5-year cutoff, by the way, is because data crunchers typically don't follow patients beyond that point.

Don't start worrying yet about whether your wife will need chemotherapy. The medical oncologist (another one of the doctors she'll have to see) will make that determination, based on tumor size, lymph node involvement, and other factors. "We need to wait until we find out more," Dr. Brennecke tells her newly diagnosed patients.

You will indeed find out a lot more. As the weeks and months go by, your wife will be bombarded with information about tumor size, cancer types, lymph node involvement, estrogen receptivity, white blood cell counts, and many other topics. One of you might want to buy a loose-leaf binder and a hole puncher, and start compiling all the doctor's reports (not to mention the stream of bills) that will come into your life. When Katy Kelly and Steve Bottorf of Washington, D.C., were done with their breast cancer binder, filling it with documents about her lumpectomy, her chemotherapy, and her radiation, it was 3½ inches thick and weighed 4 pounds.

RULES FOR COPING

I did, as you may have guessed, make amends for my slow start as a breast cancer husband. I started going to every appointment, and I found there's much a husband can do for his wife. But I can't say I was enjoying my new career. Every time it seemed that Marsha and I thought we knew what was going on, we'd get an unpleasant surprise—like the second cancerous lump. When we got that news, I could feel my last reserves of optimism draining away. Breast cancer was running—and ruining—our lives.

In short, I felt like a victim. And I hated that feeling. I hated it so much that I remember standing in my office one afternoon and saying to myself, "I'm not going to be a victim anymore." I can't tell you exactly how to make this leap—it's mind over matter, I suppose. But by all means, go ahead and try.

When I faltered in my resolve, I gained strength from an article I came across by Randy Markey, a Boston-area psychotherapist and writer who is in the thick of a lifelong fight against hydrocephalus, fluid on the brain. I e-mailed him to tell him how moved I was by an essay he wrote for our local paper. His reply gave me the fortitude to carry on: "My experiences have been like the beginning of *ABC's Wide World of Sports,* the thrill of victory and the agony of defeat. So long as doctors and I can recognize together, *together,* that we are both human, and that when we fight together, the disease process is bested whether we win or lose, then everyone wins no matter the outcome."

Marc Heyison of Rockville, Maryland, who founded the group Men Against Breast Cancer after his mother's ordeal with the disease, also seeks to inspire with a sports image. When he speaks to audiences about his educational and fund-raising organization, he likes to borrow the words of the immortal Vince Lombardi, "It's not whether you get knocked down, it's whether you get up." Once the breast cancer husband gets back up, he's got plenty of work ahead of him. And not just as a caregiver.

The trials and tribulations of daily life go on . . . and on . . . and on. In the weeks after my wife was diagnosed, we were frantically planning a bat mitzvah, helping our younger daughter cope with the first weeks of middle

---

WHAT HAPPENS WHEN

Your wife's just been diagnosed with breast cancer. What next? As she runs from doctor to doctor, she may not get a clear picture of how her treatments will progress. Here's how it usually goes.

Surgery: The initial treatment, unless docs want to shrink the tumor with chemo. Doctors like to cut out the tumor within a month of diagnosis—sooner if your wife has a particularly aggressive cancer or rare (and rapidly spreading) inflammatory breast cancer.

Reconstruction: Can be done at the same time as the mastectomy for early-stage patients, but it's your wife's choice.

Chemotherapy: Typically the second treatment, commencing a few weeks (or more) after surgery, when your wife has recovered from the removal of the lump or of her breast.

Radiation: Often the third (and final) stage of active treatment. Sometimes radiation is given along with chemo, depending on the mix of chemo drugs.

Hormonal therapies: When "active" treatment ends, your wife may take antiestrogen medications.

school (she came home in tears the first day, overwhelmed by the parade of teachers with all their rules and pet peeves), running her to the emergency room at midnight after she fractured her wrist at a roller skating party, and dragging our cat to the vet to treat a mysterious puncture wound. ("We may have to put in a drain," the veterinarian said, to which I wanted to reply, "Hold it right there, doc—because my wife's already got one!")

And, oh yes, trying to keep up with our jobs, and figuring out how we'd manage to pay the bills after my employer cut my salary by 10 percent because of the economic downturn. Why do bad things happen to breast cancer couples? I felt as if I were walking around with a big plate balanced on one hand, and people kept dumping more stuff on it. At what point, I wondered, would I drop the plate? What I found (and what others have told me) is that the human spirit is resilient, and somehow you will find the strength to carry on.

Besides, no matter what is happening to you, there's always someone else who's suffering more. Four years ago, John Salamone of Alexandria, Virginia, who was 31 years old at the time, went through open-heart surgery for a congenital defect. Six weeks later, the day before her 30th birthday, his wife, Jeanine, was diagnosed with breast cancer. "I went in our bedroom and lay on the bed and screamed as loud as I could," John says. "I was just devastated."

If you're really feeling sorry for yourself, think about the trials and tribulations of Jim Hall of Draper, Utah. Four years ago, his wife, Michelle, was diagnosed with breast cancer at age 33. She had a mastectomy and was treated with chemotherapy and radiation. The software development firm Jim worked for ran out of cash (although Jim kept working without a salary for 6 months because his employer was carrying his health insurance). In the middle of Michelle's chemo, the couple's 4-year-old daughter, who has mild cerebral palsy, suffered a seizure and had to be taken by helicopter to a hospital that could provide proper care. Then Jim and his dad went on a fishing trip in Idaho, and his dad missed a step on the stairs, fell, broke his back, and died 7 days later.

"Oh man, that just sucked along with cancer and all that crap," Jim says.

A cousin—whose new cat had just died—tried to say she knew how Jim and Michelle felt because of her pet's demise.

"We were like, you've got to be friggin' kidding me," Jim says.

"Still angry?" I ask.

"Ya think?" Jim answers, and laughs.

ANGER MANAGEMENT

Which brings me to another point. People will say—and ask—all sorts of things about your wife's cancer. No one would ask you how much money you earn or how often you have sex—but good friends, casual acquaintances, and coworkers might want to know which breast it is, and did they catch it early, and did her hair fall out, and all sorts of other intimate details.

When one husband heard the "did they catch it early" question one time too many, he snapped back, "Nope, it's too late. Do you know anybody you can fix me up with?"

Perhaps he was a tad harsh. But Roz Kleban understands what he was thinking. As administrative supervisor of social work services at the Memorial Sloan-Kettering Cancer Center in New York City, she runs support groups for breast cancer patients, as well as a group for husbands of patients undergoing chemotherapy. This particular husband's wife had been diagnosed with early-stage breast cancer, she says, but he was trying to show the questioner what a hole he was stepping into by asking such a question. What if they hadn't caught it early?

"If you're inclined," Kleban says, "you can be polite and educative" when asked about your wife's breast cancer. If it's helpful for you to talk about the details of the disease, then go ahead and talk. If not, stop the conversation. You have every right to say, "I don't feel like talking about that now." If a question ticks you off, you might choose to reply, "It's none of your business," or "Gee, what an inappropriate question." Or just change the subject.

Even if your style is not to lash out at a misguided questioner, you may find that you have a lot of anger lurking within. And sometimes it just has to come out. But try to channel your anger productively. I plead guilty to sometimes losing it when on the phone with a clueless clerk or a heartless bureaucrat, and even though I know that yelling doesn't necessarily get results, it felt good.

Some men (and their wives) look for a culprit for the disease—who's responsible for this breast cancer, anyway? My advice: Don't play the blame game. It may be true that a doctor didn't read a mammogram correctly in the past or may have missed some telltale sign. If you believe you have grounds for a lawsuit, you should contact a lawyer who specializes in medical malpractice as soon as you can. Each state has its own time limit on such suits, and the clock starts ticking at diagnosis.

Otherwise, try to look forward, not backward. If a doctor is making your wife mad—by being uncommunicative or unsympathetic—then the best thing you can do is to help her find another doctor. And if the medical bureaucracy is getting you down, at least you and your wife have each other. "It was us against the world, against those doctors who didn't give us results right away, those clerks who couldn't find the mammogram," says Neal Engledow, 56, of Centreville, Virginia, whose wife, Ganga Jali Engledow, 54, was diagnosed 2 years ago.

If your wife is blaming herself for causing her own breast cancer, you should tell her what doctor after doctor told me. "When women ask, 'Why did I get this—was it my diet or whatever?' I tell them, 'We don't know what causes breast cancer,'" says breast surgeon Katherine Alley, M.D., medical director of the Suburban Breast Center in Bethesda, Maryland.

Once your wife has assembled a good team of doctors and they've advised her on a treatment plan, some of your anger and free-floating anxiety will disappear—to be replaced by specific anxieties. Such as: How will the surgery go? What's chemo like? Radiation—does that mean my wife will be radioactive?

I hope I can give you the answers to these questions as you read on, even if the answer will sometimes be, "It depends."

HAVE FUN

Another way to offset your anger is to have fun. I mean it. Those are two of the most important words I can pass on to you.

You might well be wondering how to have fun in the face of a life-threatening disease—and an overwhelmingly complicated one at that. "Breast cancer is an anomaly among cancers," warns psychologist Julia Rowland,

Ph.D., who runs the Office of Cancer Survivorship at the National Cancer Institute in Bethesda, Maryland. There's no one-cure-fits-all treatment. Just about every time your wife has to make a decision, she'll have two—or three or four—choices. And there won't necessarily be a right answer. Her decision will rest upon many different elements—the nature of her tumor, but also her doctor's advice and her own preferences. And she must make these decisions at a time when she is at the peak of emotional vulnerability, still reeling from the news that she has cancer.

"You've been hit by a train, and it's just the beginning of the train," says Susan Abrams, a Maryland oncological social worker who has been counseling women with cancer for 30 years. "It's like having an out-of-body experience. Even when you are acting normally, asking questions, doing what you need to do, collecting your information—part of you is there and part of you isn't."

Being hit by a train, well, that's not much fun at all.

After the train comes the roller coaster. That's the image many breast cancer couples use to describe their experience. It's apt in many ways: They're up, they're down, they're dizzy, their hearts are in their throats, and they have a sick feeling in the pit of their stomachs. But the point of an amusement park roller coaster is to have fun—and the ride usually doesn't last more than 2 minutes. The breast cancer roller coaster, however, seems to be devoid of enjoyment—and there's no end in sight. Your wife will face the surgeon's knife, and possibly the oncologist's chemicals, and the radiation oncologist's x-rays, not to mention myriad unforeseen complications that could crop up. If your wife is going to have all three treatments, then the two of you are looking at nearly a year of fighting cancer, from the moment of diagnosis to the time, a few months after treatment ends, when she begins to feel like herself again. "I always considered that year to be a sacrifice you make in the interest of the rest of your life," says surgeon Sherwin Nuland, M.D., author of the extraordinarily moving (and award-winning) *How We Die: Reflections on Life's Final Chapter.* "'Investment' is probably a better word."

There you are, stuck on the world's least enjoyable roller coaster. "I used up 50 years of reserve emotion in the first week," one husband confessed.

So, where's the fun? Separately and together, you and your wife need to do things that help you rebuild your energy supplies. In other words, fun things—whether it's taking in a movie, going on a hike, or playing a round of golf. (A word to the wise: Don't schedule the golf game for the day of the biopsy.)

Inch by inch, fun crept back into our lives, and we were glad to see it.

One of the best times to have fun were the "limbo days"—that's what we came to call those stretches when Marsha was waiting for test results or a second opinion, so she couldn't do anything about the cancer. On limbo days, all we could do was to be parents, and employees, and lovers, and friends. Just like we used to be before breast cancer.

Your natural inclination might be to fret, but you'll be much better off if you can use those precious hours in the pursuit of happiness. I remember fondly a delicious carryout Chinese dinner, an evening watching a mindless video, a half-hour's walk admiring the sunset. As preposterous as it might sound, egg rolls and an evening stroll can temporarily put cancer at bay.

TIPS ➢ ➢ ➢

1. A needle biopsy is becoming the standard of care, although there may be reasons for a surgical biopsy (the location of the tumor, for one). Ask the doctor to explain the choice of biopsy procedure.
2. Grab any time you can to relax with your wife—a hike, a movie, dinner out. You'll be grateful for the respite from cancer.
3. Avoid looking back and asking, "How did this cancer happen?" Doing so isn't going to help as you try to move forward with a treatment plan.

➢ BONUS TIP

If you buy your wife self-help books, pick up at least one about life after breast cancer. That's what Chris Rippie of Bear, Delaware, did for his fiancée Debra Wood. "That was wonderful," she says. "It let me know that yes, you're going through it, but these people went through it and look at them. It's not a death sentence." A fine choice: *After Breast Cancer: A Common-Sense Guide to Life After Treatment* by Hester Hill Schnipper, oncological social worker and breast cancer survivor.

Do Men Walk Out?

Most don't, but there is more than one way to abandon your wife

I'm at a breast cancer workshop that's part of the Susan G. Komen Breast Cancer Foundation's annual mission conference. The topic is "Communicating with People After Diagnosis." The hotel meeting room is packed with dozens of breast cancer survivors. I ask a question, and I mention that I'm working on a book about breast cancer husbands.

A trim, 40-ish woman on the other side of the room pops up from her seat. Dressed in sparkly sweats, she has a good-natured expression and short-cropped, blond-streaked hair. "What about the men who leave their wives?" she demands.

A chorus of backup voices chimes in: "Yeah, what about 'em?" Just like the die-hard fans who yell, "Throw the bum out!" at a baseball game.

To tell the truth, I was not surprised by the response.

HALL OF SHAMEFUL HUSBANDS

It seems as if just about everyone has a story to share about a bad breast cancer husband. A breast surgeon told me about a feckless fellow who abandoned his wife and two young children, leaving her to face chemo (and care for the kids) on her own. Another spouse took his wife back to her mother, as if she were a defective piece of merchandise, and announced, "I can't deal with this."

At the Y-ME hotline, a breast cancer survivor called up one day and said, "I'm in the middle of making dinner for my husband, but I don't know why, because he's having an affair."

Hotline volunteer counselor Sandee Stern of Chicago, a breast cancer survivor, asked, "Does he know that you know?"

"He told me," the caller replied. "And he said he won't break it off because if something happens to me, he doesn't want to be alone."

Longtime boyfriends can behave just as reprehensibly. "He related my breast cancer to a root canal. A root canal!" says a 50-year-old woman who participated in a breast cancer study run by sociologist Saskia Subramanian at the UCLA Center for Culture and Health. "That was real, real hurtful. Later on, I found out that he had moved some other lady in with him."

I guess those guys are trying to stoop to the level of Newt Gingrich. The former Speaker of the House of Representatives visited his estranged wife, Jackie, in the hospital after she was recuperating from surgery for uterine cancer and reportedly asked her to sign a hand-drafted divorce document. (At least that's what she said; he denied that he did such a dastardly deed.)

When I hear such accounts, I begin to wonder if men lack an empathy gene. That idea isn't as far-fetched as it sounds. Karen Weihs, M.D., a psychiatrist who studies cancer and families at George Washington University in Washington, D.C., believes that women are certainly socialized to be more empathetic than men. Women may have a biological edge in the empathy department, too. They secrete lots of oxytocin when giving birth, nursing a baby, or making love. Researchers believe this hormone encourages nurturing behavior in women; they haven't determined if men get the same empathy-boost from the oxytocin they produce. That doesn't mean a guy can't learn. But it might take a little practice to get it right. The chapter Your Wife's Feelings on page 48 can help get you started.

The tales of rogue breast cancer husbands are bad enough. To make matters worse, lots of people seem to believe there's an honest-to-goodness academic study proving that breast cancer couples split up at a higher rate than couples in the general population. And that would have to be a pretty high rate indeed, since one out of every two marriages ends in divorce. "For breast cancer to have an effect that would be measurable," says Julia Rowland, Ph.D., the National Cancer Institute psychologist, "It would have to be a whopping effect."

Perhaps folks are recalling a study about cancer and divorce that made the rounds 3 years ago, garnering headlines on CNN and other news outlets. Mike Glantz, M.D., presented the data at the American Society of Clinical Oncology. An associate professor at the University of Massachusetts School of Medicine in Worcester, Dr. Glantz is a neuro-oncologist—that means he treats patients with brain tumors. In his practice, he noticed a certain number of divorces among patients in the time from diagnosis to death, so he began keeping track. He looked at 214 couples where one partner had a terminal

BREAST CANCER SAVED THEIR MARRIAGE

"At one point, it looked like breast cancer was going to drive us completely apart," says Bobbye Sloan, wife of Jerry Sloan, the Utah Jazz basketball coach. Instead, it brought Bobbye and Jerry back together again.

The two have been a couple for 3 decades, since they were high school sweethearts in Illinois. But when Bobbye was diagnosed 7 years ago at age 54, they were leading separate lives. "NBA life is tough on a marriage," she says. "We had a long period when he just went his way and I went my way."

Bobbye didn't tell Jerry about her breast cancer diagnosis until after her mastectomy. He'd left Utah for their Illinois summer home. She said she was staying on in Salt Lake City for a previously scheduled surgical procedure, and didn't mention that she had another surgery on the docket. "He doesn't deal with illness very well," she explains. She knew he'd react with doom and gloom, and she didn't want any of that. "I don't want to wake up after surgery and see his sad, sorry face," she thought. "I'm just gonna get through this as best as I can."

Before chemo began, Bobbye told her husband what was going on. But Jerry didn't rally to the cause. Bobbye had to postpone her last infusion because her white blood cell counts were so low. "I was just beat," she says. Meanwhile, Jerry was "living the life he brain tumor. Twenty-three of the couples divorced. In 18 cases, it was the man who left his fatally ill spouse. In five instances, the woman walked out on a dying husband. CNN used this misleading headline to characterize the study: "Divorce rate higher for terminal cancer patients."

"We can't speak to whether the rate of divorce is greater than, less than, or equal to the rate in the general population," Dr. Glantz says. And he stresses that "it's not the majority of men who are leaving." Cancer experts agree. "I think men are very decent human beings," says Matthew Loscalzo, who is the director of patient and family support services at the University of California at San Diego Cancer Center. In his years of counseling cancer couples, he has seen no evidence of a mass exodus by men.

Nonetheless, Dr. Glantz was struck by the asymmetry he uncovered. In

---

had been before," she says. "It entailed a lot of alcohol." He came in from a late-night outing, and she poured out her heart: "Here I am fighting for my life, and you're snuffing yours out.

"He just kind of stomped around the next day," she says. "And he said, 'You know what? I'm going to make some changes. Let's see if we can't get this back on track.'"

Jerry was a man of his word. "Our marriage was not the best in the world at that particular time," he says. "I'd been drinking too much. I quit that. I quit smoking, too. Our whole life changed."

"We started our lives over again," Bobbye agrees. "Our love is stronger than it ever was. Sometimes when you're faced with the possibility of losing someone you love, you look at the situation through different eyes."

"Basketball doesn't really mean anything," says Jerry. "It's just a way to make a living." He laughs, because it's clearly still much more than that to him. But it's not his end-all and be-all. He takes time for the little things—like admiring the birds that fly over his country home ("I knew they were out there, but I didn't know which was which") and admiring the woman who bravely faced her breast cancer. "As far as our life is concerned," he says, "it's never been better."

his sampling, men were more likely to walk out on an afflicted spouse than were women in the same situation.

Surely a terminal brain tumor presents a different set of conditions than a diagnosis of breast cancer. So Dr. Glantz looked at the divorce rate among a group of 193 general oncology patients: 107 women and 86 men. Nearly two-thirds of the women had been diagnosed with breast cancer. By Dr. Glantz's count, 13 men walked out on a wife diagnosed with cancer, but only one woman left a cancer-stricken husband.

Dr. Glantz's study has been submitted for publication but has not yet been peer reviewed and published. So at this point, it represents one doctor's carefully vetted slice of life. His possible explanation of his findings: "In our culture, men aren't accustomed, aren't trained, aren't exposed to being the primary caregiver in the setting of a devastating illness." His hope is to establish ways to help men who are floundering in this unfamiliar role.

Meanwhile, husbands and wives can take heart from a Canadian study. "Marital Stability After Breast Cancer," which appeared in the *Journal of the National Cancer Institute* in January 1999, addresses the "belief that husbands desert wives who have breast cancer," says coauthor Jill Taylor-Brown, who is director of psychosocial oncology and supportive care at CancerCare Manitoba. The authors of the study examined data that had been previously compiled on two groups of women of similar ages from Quebec City: 200 women who were newly diagnosed with non-metastatic breast cancer, and two other randomly selected groups of married Quebec City women. So this wasn't just a report on how breast cancer patients fared; it compared them with the general population. The breast cancer patients answered questions about how their relationship with their spouse seemed 3 months after diagnosis, 18 months after diagnosis, then 8 years after diagnosis. The choices ranged from "very unsatisfactory" to "perfectly happy." The women who did not have breast cancer answered similar questions about "degree of happiness" with their spouse.

The result: almost a tie. In both groups, around three couples out of 100 divorced or separated. The rate of women reporting "marital dissatisfaction" was also about the same—on average, around 1 in 10. As you might expect, the breast cancer patients who complained of poor marital satisfaction 3 months after diagnosis were the ones most likely to suffer further strains in their relationship. "For the times studied," the authors conclude, "breast cancer does not appear to be associated with marital breakdown among Quebec women." The study is well known among mental health professionals who follow breast cancer, but somehow the message hasn't made it to the rest of the world.

Doctors and therapists have found that their real-life observations match the results of the study. In their experience, the majority of husbands stand by their wives. "Most husbands are good guys," says Hester Hill Schnipper, chief of oncology social work at Boston's Beth Israel Deaconess Medical Center and herself a breast cancer survivor. "They love their wives, and they're scared to death along with them."

Those loyal husbands are ticked off by the very thought of the heartless cancer husband. "Whenever I talk to husbands about this issue," says Taylor-Brown, "many of them feel insulted that anyone would think they'd leave their wife at a time like this. Their reaction is, 'What kind of a jerk do you think I am that I'd do such a thing?'"

That's what Jonathan Davis of Boston found himself thinking last year, after his wife was diagnosed with cancer. In a down moment during her treatment for breast cancer, Michele said to him, "You should leave me and find somebody who's whole." Jonathan, 46, had no intention of leaving. But Michele's statement made him wonder how anyone could, in fact, walk out. "I couldn't face myself if I did. How could you do that? Even if things had been awful and we were unhappy, I would think in a crisis a husband would put off those feelings."

THE REAL WORLD

Of course, any study represents only a slice of life. The reality of breast cancer is that it is a complex disease, and it will almost surely have a profound effect on your marriage, for better or worse. "Cancer magnifies imperfections in any relationship," says oncologist Fred Smith, M.D., who practices in Chevy Chase, Maryland. Even the best relationship has its share of imperfections. And I don't have to tell you that no husband is perfect.

The first flash point is the moment of diagnosis. As I've already confessed,

GUY TALK

"Some men feel they can't handle a wife's breast cancer and just bail out. But I mean, this is your wife. How are you gonna bail out at the time she needs you the most? I married her because I love her, because I want to be with her. You gotta be a man and deal with it."

—EDWIN COTTO, 43
Garfield, New Jersey

I didn't exactly get off on the right foot. Okay, I was 100 percent on the wrong foot. Instead of rushing home to my wife's side when she called me at the office with news of a tentative diagnosis, I mumbled a few noncommittal words and stayed at work.

I figured that when I told my story to therapists, they'd call me a cad. What I learned instead is that my initial reaction was a normal response to distressing medical news about a spouse. "Who wants to hear that?" says Venus Masselam, Ph.D., a psychologist in Bethesda, Maryland, who has counseled numerous breast cancer patients over the years, and who tells it like it is when it comes to the disease and its impact on a couple. "Your instinct is not to want to believe it—'Ooh, it's not really true.' Because you don't want to believe." You don't want to face the reality that your wife has breast cancer and that your lives will be altered in ways large and small.

"Men may push away," notes Dr. Smith, "to steel themselves from any perceived loss to come." That could be the beginning of the end of a marriage—unless the husband moves past his initial wave of panic.

A woman in the same situation might feel the same way. "I don't know any woman who says, 'I can't wait for my husband to have prostate cancer so I can be there for him,'" Dr. Masselam says. "It goes against human nature to want to be burdened with anyone."

You *can* make amends for a rough start, but not if you remain in denial. And certainly not if your selfishness overwhelms your selflessness. "There are husbands who don't want to hear about this," says Robert Siegel, M.D., the director of hematology and oncology at George Washington University Medical Faculty Associates in Washington, D.C. "They want a sexual partner. This is not what they bargained for when they got married."

Indeed. A friend told me about a newlywed who asked his just-diagnosed wife if she might defer her mastectomy until sailing season was over. She pitched that loser overboard.

When I tell women about the sailing husband, they tend to say something like, "Thank God she found out what a schmuck he was before they had kids." In other words, maybe some of these bad breast cancer husbands were just plain bad husbands. And one thing you can count on: The diagnosis of a life-threatening illness isn't likely to make your past troubles disappear. The Komen conference woman who asked about husbands who walk out—it turns out that her husband vanished from the scene after her diagnosis. But she also told me that he had a substance abuse problem before her cancer and was clearly spiraling downward. They eventually divorced, and she went out and found a new boyfriend.

But it's impossible to predict how breast cancer will affect a relationship. Some couples who weren't especially close before the diagnosis are able to pull together to fight the cancer as a team. Conversely, some marriages that seemed to be working just fine suddenly take a tumble. What's more, a husband doesn't have to walk out the door to abandon his wife.

ANOTHER WAY TO WALK OUT

Regal and serene, Della Franklin* is a woman who knows how to get what she needs. Because she had polio as a child, she uses a wheelchair, but she maneuvers with dignity and determination. At the plush hotel restaurant where we had lunch, she pow-wowed with the hostess to get the table she wanted, then deftly steered her chair through the narrow spaces in the restaurant, politely asking seated diners to give her a little more room when she needed it.

But when she was diagnosed with breast cancer ("like being hit by a Mack truck," she recalled) and had to endure a mastectomy and chemotherapy, she did not get what she needed from her husband.

"His initial reaction was kind of sympathetic," remembered Della, 56, a federal employee in Washington, D.C. But then, as often happens with breast cancer, things didn't proceed smoothly. She had complications from her mastectomy. She suffered panic attacks. She grew depressed. "I was frightened shitless," she said. She thought her husband was frightened, too, and that he probably felt she was falling apart right before his eyes. His body language told her that he didn't want to be by her side at doctor's appointments.

What *did* she want him to do?

The restaurant had grown quiet as the lunch crowd dispersed. In our hushed corner of the nearly empty eatery, Della paused, then said one word.

"Listen."

It's that simple. And it's that hard.

She let the word hang there for a minute, because that's the word all of us breast cancer husbands should wear on a chain around our necks.

Then she continued: "You need to be able to talk with somebody. When that somebody is a husband, I believe it's got to be one of the most bonding experiences that can go on."

And then Della issued another command: "Don't belittle. One thing a husband should avoid is passing on the message that you're not handling it well, that you are a wimp, that you're a flake. Because you know what? Some days you are stronger than others. And on your weak days, what you really want is for someone to say, 'I know this is bad, but it's all right. Just hang on, because tomorrow's going to be better, and I'm going to be there for you tomorrow.' I didn't want someone to engage in a pity party with me. But I wanted someone to say, 'Hey, you know what? You're a trouper. I know you don't feel strong now, but you're gonna be stronger down the pike.'"

Five years after her treatment, Della and her husband are still together. She's made her peace with the past. "If you harbor anger and allow it to fester, it does you so much harm," she explains. "The Lord has enabled me to turn it loose." When her husband faced prostate cancer a few months after her diagnosis, he began to understand what she had been through.

But for Nora Lane*, the story doesn't have quite as happy an ending.

Soft-spoken and thoughtful, 57-year-old Nora has a warm smile and a down-to-earth style of dressing. When she was diagnosed with cancer 3 years ago, she and her husband had just relocated to Chicago, where he had taken a job. She was starting to search for work. The diagnosis ended her job hunt—and began a disturbing new phase in their marriage. At a chemotherapy planning session, her husband asked to speak to the oncologist alone. She later learned from the doctor that her husband had complained that she was too preoccupied with her "cancer problem." He had hoped the doctor would tell Nora to start job-hunting, because surely work would "distract" her during treatment. The oncologist told her husband the suggestion was inappropriate, which he wasn't happy to hear.

Nora didn't look for a job. And her husband never went along to another doctor's appointment. She had a bad reaction to her first chemo treatment. Her husband panicked—and began a disappearing act. He left home in the morning before she awoke, worked late, and went to bed as soon as he got home. "I really didn't need physical care," Nora says. "I didn't need anyone to watch me or feed me, the way someone who has a stroke needs care." All she wanted was a little kindness, a carryout dinner from time to time, and a back rub when she couldn't sleep. "If men only realized how even little attentions from them will get an enormous return," she says wistfully.

"I think he's uncomfortable with some of his feelings," she says, trying to figure out what went wrong. "He's a man. He doesn't have close friends to speak to. He's also very smart. So he knows he could do better, and that makes him feel worse."

They've tried therapy. The therapist suggested that her husband's behavior was a result of fear that he'd lose Nora. Yet he pretty much has, because of the way he's acting. Go figure.

Now they live in limbo. Her husband is holed up in his study. Nora has asked him flat out: "Do you want a divorce? Do you want to separate?"

She can't get a straight answer.

She's beginning to set deadlines in her mind, because she doesn't want to live the rest of her life this way.

And she's haunted by the memory of a breast cancer workshop at a local hospital. The therapist leading the group asked, "How do men respond to breast cancer?" A husband raised his hand and said, "Men leave."

"My husband didn't leave me," Nora says. "But emotionally, he did."

A HUSBAND'S ADVICE

Men aren't the only ones who walk out after a breast cancer diagnosis. Perhaps the things you say and do (or don't say and do) will cause your wife to walk out on you.

"You're not going to want to hear what I have to say," a 50-something breast cancer survivor told me as we chatted on an Avon breast cancer walk in Boston. When she was going through chemotherapy, her husband didn't like the fact that she was sick. He wasn't there for her. After she finished treatment, she wasn't there for him. She filed for divorce, quit her job, and went back to college to become a guidance counselor. Striding purposefully along Boston's streets on a brisk and sunny spring day, she looked wonderful—full of vitality and purpose and confidence.

Now there's a lesson for all breast cancer husbands: If we're not with the program, we may not be *on* the program.

Which is not to say it's easy to be a breast cancer husband. Jeffrey Berger remembers those moments of doubt after his wife's diagnosis: "Am I going to freak out, or fall apart, or not handle it well?" He found strength in a quote from the Rev. Dr. Martin Luther King, Jr.: "The ultimate measure of a man is not where he stands in moments of comfort and convenience, but where he stands at times of challenge and controversy." Breast cancer was "a true test of our relationship," Jeffrey says. "And I think it's gotten better. We have cheated death. When something else comes up, we say, 'Pfft, this is nothing.'"

And really, all it takes is love and understanding. At an exceedingly damp Race for the Cure in Washington, D.C., last year, I struck up a conversation with Doug and Nancy Ayers of Fairfax, Virginia. He's 66 and she's 61—and 20 years out from her breast cancer diagnosis. I asked Doug if he has any words of wisdom for all of us new breast cancer husbands. "You just hug and kiss her," he said. A wave of emotion washed over his face as he spoke. He might have shed a few tears, but it was hard to tell because of the downpour. Then he heeded his own advice, drawing Nancy close for a passionate, rain-soaked kiss.

TIPS ➢ ➢ ➢

1. Don't be scared by stories of men who flee because they can't cope. Most marriages survive. Some even thrive.
2. Repeat after me: "I understand how you feel, dear." Now say it like you mean it. The more you practice empathy, experts say, the more empathetic you are likely to become.
3. If your marriage had "issues" before breast cancer, the problems aren't going to disappear. A few sessions with a therapist might be in order.

➢ BONUS TIP

Your wife might say (darkly) that you should leave her and find someone else. You can respond with an affectionate declaration of love or with humor, if that's your style. ("Nope, then I'd be just like Newt Gingrich," one husband said.) "But if the man is distressed or confused by the statement, he should say so," says psychologist Julia Rowland, Ph.D., of the Office of Cancer Survivorship of the National Cancer Institute in Bethesda, Maryland. Then the two of you should talk so you can understand what your wife means. Is she seeking a sign of your commitment? Or, if she fears that her death is likely, is she trying to give you permission to find a loving partner after she is gone?

Caregiving 101

A practical guide for clueless guys

What kind of caregivers do men make?

That was the question posed to eight breast cancer couples in a focus group at Johns Hopkins Hospital in Baltimore. The women graded their husbands on their caregiving performance during the months of diagnosis and treatment. The husbands graded themselves as well. To a man, the guys gave themselves lower grades than did their wives, who praised their husbands for their wonderful support. The men were genuinely surprised by the high marks.

So there you have it: proof that we breast cancer husbands aren't quite as bad at caring for our wives as we might think we are. "I don't think men are crummy caregivers," agrees social worker Matthew Loscalzo, director of patient and family support services at the University of California at San Diego Cancer Center, who has worked with cancer patients for over two decades and who helped run the focus group. "I think men give caring the way men give caring, and women give it in a different way."

What the breast cancer husband must learn is to be the kind of caregiver that his wife needs. "It's not about you, ya bastard," says Sherwin Nuland, M.D., with a wink. He's clinical professor of surgery at Yale University and author of the award-winning book, *How We Die*. "It's not about how *sensitive* or how *strong* you can be."

So what *is* it about? A breast cancer husband has to figure out what his wife needs from him. For years, you may have skated by with sex, Saturday nights out, and the occasional box of candy. Now you'll need to come to a deeper level of understanding. Mind reading is not recommended. Nor will renting the movie *What Women Want* give you a clue, especially in the wake of breast cancer. You may stumble along the way. "I'm sure I didn't do some things right," says Claude Robinson, 72, of Capitol Heights, Maryland, whose wife, Lawanna, underwent a lumpectomy, followed by radiation. "I just hope I did most of the things right. It's like a marriage—you don't do everything right, do you?"

Take heart—it's not an impossible job. And your wife will deeply appreciate your efforts. "Greg was my prince," says Heidi LaFleche of her husband, Greg Passler. "He rose to the occasion in ways big and small, from camping out with me in the living room [she slept on the couch because it was closer to the bathroom] to going to the pharmacy at 3:00 in the morning. He was present on every level." And he never even let on that sleeping on a worn-out futon mattress was a pain in the back.

MR. DON'T-FIX-IT

There's a lot of confusion in the male brain about what it means to be a caregiver. That's understandable. In many couples, the woman assumes more of the caregiving responsibilities. "Men are just not taught to be caregivers in any sense of that word," says social worker Jim Zabora.

Ain't that the truth. And at a time in our lives when we do need to give care—when our wives are about to give birth—at least we get a little training. When our honey is heavy with child, we dutifully accompany her to childbirth classes and learn all about the father-to-be's Very Important Job: tell the Mrs. to breathe and relax during labor. You know, just in case all those doctors and nurses forget to remind her.

Zabora is one of the many folks in the health-care field who'd like to see an educational session or two for newly diagnosed women—and for their husbands or boyfriends. Someday, that may be the norm. The Centers for Disease Control and Prevention recently awarded a $1.1 million grant to Men

Against Breast Cancer, a fund-raising and educational group based in Rockville, Maryland, to establish such programs on a pilot basis for the "underserved African-American, Latino, and Indian populations."

But right now, most men are on their own when it comes to cancer caregiving. They may mean well, but they tend to jump to the wrong conclusions. And the number one wrong conclusion: They think a caregiver has to fix things.

I don't know whether Mr. Fix-It is hardwired into our genes or drummed into our skulls, but this is one stereotype that holds true across the board. Psychologists, social workers, medical doctors, breast cancer survivors, and, of course, breast cancer husbands all agree. Guys feel compelled to "fix" cancer. We want to take it on at the basketball hoop, one on one. We want to pull out a six-shooter and start firing away. Perhaps that's why we judge ourselves harshly as cancer caregivers. No husband can defeat cancer. Ergo, we've failed to protect our wives.

That sense of powerlessness can make a husband miserable.

"My entire life revolves around fixing issues," says Colton Young, 42, who's vice president of an environmental management company outside of Philadelphia. "I get paid to go in and mitigate people's problems." When his wife, Kathleen McCarthy, was diagnosed with cancer at age 36, he had to face the fact that he couldn't fix it: "There ain't a damn thing you can do about it but sit back and hope the people you have on your team are with you. It's a horrible feeling of utter helplessness."

Paul Byers, a journalism professor from Washington, D.C., whose wife, Fran, was diagnosed with breast cancer, is familiar with the feeling. "I can do chores, I can make life easier in other ways. But I can't take on the real issue itself."

"You can't find the solution or rescue the fair maiden," agrees Carol Stevenson, 56, of Arlington, Virginia, a 4-year breast cancer survivor. But that doesn't mean the spouse is indeed helpless. Carol needed her husband, Phil Gay, to be there with her. Not to solve her problems or to conquer cancer, but to stand by her side and to accept her as she was. "The most important thing for me was to know it was all right to be sick, and not beautiful, and not the epitome of femininity. He was always there to hold me if I needed to be held or to talk to me if I needed to talk. I was very grateful for that."

GUY TALK

"Men are fighters. We want to go out and pick up a gun and shoot breast cancer. But the biggest thing men need to do is show that we care."

—STEPHEN PECK, 59
Washington, D.C., who lost his wife, Gayle, to breast cancer

Carol remembers coming home from the hospital with "bulbs and things" hanging from her armpit incision and feeling as if she were a weird-looking Christmas tree. "It was gross," she says. "But Phil accepted that, and arranged the tubes and bulbs and cuddled up next to me." That was what she needed. Not advice, not a miracle, not a Mr. Fix-It. "Just a witness" to what she was going through.

A witness—not a judge. David Kupfer of Arlington, Virginia, recalls how his fiancée, Cathy Hainer, liked to rest on the couch in the living room after chemo. That bothered him. "I wanted her to sit up or to lie on a bed upstairs," he says. "I had to work to realize that's how she wanted to be."

David had other caregiver lessons to learn. One time after Cathy's chemo, David's son (from a previous marriage) had soccer practice. He said to Cathy, "Since you are going to sleep, is it okay if I watch soccer practice?" And she said, "Sure."

Silly as it may seem, that bothered David. It bothered him that he wasn't so important that he had to be by Cathy's side every second of the day. "I had to learn that I wasn't indispensable," he says, "which really irritated me."

In other words, he had to learn that the caregiver isn't in charge—the patient is.

INDEPENDENT WOMEN

Your wife, meanwhile, may have a difficult time switching gears from caregiver to care receiver. "Women are not used to having people take care of them," says Susan Abrams, an oncological social worker in Maryland. "They don't know how to take it."

That womanly self-sufficiency can be disastrous, as Carol Stevenson is only too happy to tell you. The evening after her first chemotherapy treatment, she ate a light dinner that Phil had prepared. ("I do 80 percent of the cooking," he says. "It was no big deal for me.") A very tired Carol went to bed. Phil retreated to the den to watch a football game. He checked on her at one point, and she seemed to be asleep.

After an hour or so, he heard the toilet flush. Then he heard it flush again. The phone rang. By the time he picked it up, he could hear Carol talking to her doctor. "This isn't good," he said to himself. "She'd been sick, she was on the phone with her doctor to see if there was anything she could do about the nausea, and she decided she didn't want to bother me."

When I spoke with Phil, who's 63, it was 4 years after that night of nausea. But he remembers exactly what he said to Carol: "What am I here for? What do you think I am—a potted plant?"

Carol and Phil still joke about the potted plant moment. But it was more than just a funny line. "After that, very slowly, she was able to allow me to do things she wouldn't normally have asked me to do," says Phil. "I said, 'Don't get used to this. When it's all over, you can go back to being independent.'"

THE POWER OF LOVE

Okay, so now you know you can't fix breast cancer. But you definitely should be doing something, even if your wife isn't asking. Where do you start?

"That's the reaction I get from a lot of men," says Michael Tucker, the *L.A. Law* actor whose wife (and co-star) Jill Eikenberry was diagnosed with breast cancer when the hit TV series had just begun its run. "What's my job? What's my job?"

Start by telling your wife that you love her. These are words that are sometimes hard to say, sometimes easy to say. But no one else can say them in the same way that you can. And there's never been a better time for you to say them.

"There have actually been studies that show that women who have the support of their families do better in the long run," says Katherine Alley,

M.D., medical director of the Suburban Breast Center in Bethesda, Maryland. It's not that these women beat cancer at a higher rate. But they cope better with the anxiety and depression triggered by diagnosis, and with the crushing stress of the treatments. "I think it's the emotional support, the physical support," Dr. Alley says. "It's being able to tell a woman that 'I don't care if you lose every hair on your head, I don't care if you have to lose your breast. I don't love you for your body.' I think it's just really important to have somebody who cares, because it's not easy to go through breast cancer treatment."

What if you're not feeling love in your heart at that moment? Marriages have ups and downs, and maybe you and your wife are going through one of the downs. "This is not the time to tell your wife you don't think you love her," suggests Marisa Weiss, M.D., a Philadelphia breast radiation oncologist and founder and president of the nonprofit organization and Web site www.breastcancer.org. "A lot of times people bring up everything that was wrong for the last 10 years."

Instead of revisiting the past, consider a moratorium on the rehashing of old wounds. "Sometimes it's good for the wife to set some ground rules," Dr. Weiss says. "Okay, I know that was a bad move I made whenever, and it's okay to talk about it a little longer tonight, but after tonight, the scope of discussion is limited to the last 6 months to a year." Or else, you and your wife may find yourselves at loggerheads. She might tell you, "You're not meeting my needs, you never have." If you're the one having a meltdown (which can happen, believe me), try not to say anything you'll wind up regretting.

Instead of looking backward, look ahead. What happens during breast cancer treatment could set a new course for your marriage. Cancer "wiped the slate clean," says Heidi LaFleche. "We were starting from a new point. And Greg walked through the fire with me. He helped me choose life. I think I'm doing well today because he helped, and I hope he knows I really appreciate it."

And remember: The little things count. "That extra snuggle, holding hands at a time when you're not expecting it, the 'I love you's' make you know you are precious to this person," says TV journalist Linda Ellerbee, who underwent a bilateral mastectomy, followed by chemotherapy. "Then you don't feel so alone, because you *feel very alone* going through cancer."

THE JOB LIST

Caregiving, as you'll see, has both an emotional and a practical side to it. Some husbands are good at figuring out the latter. Others need help.

Here's a hint from social worker Matthew Loscalzo about what you might say to your wife as you embark on your caregiving career: "We all know that men need a mission, and my new mission is to be there for you in any way I can. But I don't know how to help. You have to tell me what you want. Is there anything I can do for you right now?"

But don't be a nudge. "The first thing I tell husbands," says breast cancer survivor Sandee Stern, who counsels couples on the Y-ME breast cancer hotline, "is don't push it. Do whatever she will allow you to do. Offer, but don't hover, because then you'll just get into an argument."

One thing you can offer is a back rub—something simple, and something you know you can carry off successfully. "Men are success-oriented," Michael Tucker points out. "If it's games, or work, or making love, we want to do well."

I can relate to that. I thought I'd be doing well if I could come up with the ultimate to-do list for breast cancer husbands—the top 10 things that make a difference.

Early in my research for this book, I spoke to guys who went online and who read voraciously, tracking down useful information to present to their wives. Now that seems like a role tailor-made for men. Guys are hunters by nature, right? And what wife wouldn't be grateful for the data they bag. I thought I'd found the first job for the breast cancer husband's job list: data hound.

Turns out I was wrong on several counts. "The amount of information that's good for one person is not the amount of information that somebody else needs," says Mary Ann McCabe, Ph.D., a licensed clinical psychologist and associate professor at the George Washington University School of Medicine in Washington, D.C., who has been counseling families with cancer for 15 years. Your wife may—or may not—want to hear what you've found. Furthermore, not every husband is cut out for the job. "I wanted the cancer to go away," says David Houser, 53, of Olney, Maryland, whose wife, Conny, used to read aloud to him from *Dr. Susan Love's Breast Book*. "But I felt a responsibility to know what was going on."

So if it suits you, you can be the information finder; and if it suits your wife, you can tell her what you find. The point is that at least one of you might want to research breast cancer. But whether it's you or your wife (or a family member with a medical background), the goal isn't to find a cure for the disease. "It's that you get enough information to ask the right questions," advises Dick Greenberg, whose computer-literate wife, Carla, was a Web browser.

I also figured that a guy to-do list should include handling the medical bills (and inevitable bill snafus). After all, your poor wife has enough to do just enduring the treatments. Some guys do take on this task. Then again, your wife may just be a better bill straightener-outer. That's the way it was in our household. Marsha would panic when a bill would arrive, and my job was to say, "Don't worry, honey, that must be a mistake—we can't really owe the hospital $1 million and 11 cents." Marsha, who is far better at intimidating bureaucrats than I am, would spring into action. Tough and thorough and unrelenting, she'd make the call . . . and get put on hold . . . and curse a little . . . and speak to a clerk who had not a clue . . . and ask to speak to a supervisor . . . and refuse to take no for an answer . . . and eventually she'd get the error cleared up.

Then again, maybe neither of you wants to take on the insurance dragons. I spoke to some couples who hired a medical accountant to handle this time-consuming task.

The more couples I interviewed, the more I came to see that the caregiver's job list can't be carved on stone tablets. It depends upon who you are and who your wife is, what kinds of strengths and weaknesses each of you has, and how your marriage works. It also depends on your wife's prognosis, her frame of mind, and the kinds of treatments she has to undergo—and particularly, whether she is a candidate for chemo (which I'll cover in Coping with Chemo on page 197, because chemo can be the ultimate test of a breast cancer husband's caregiving skills).

You'll need to figure out what works for you and your wife—and what to do when problems arise. Who knows, maybe you can solve them. But

(continued on page 40)

CARING FOR THE CAREGIVER

In addition to caring for your wife—and any kids you may have—you need to take care of yourself. Because frankly, if you don't, no one else will.

The idea of taking "me time" makes guys a little uneasy. Tom Stern, who talks to breast cancer husbands on the Y-ME hotline, often asks, "What do you do for yourself?" They'll say, "nothing." And he'll reply, "You have to recharge your batteries. Take 10 minutes to shoot baskets, read, ride a bike. Do it."

Ask your wife if it's okay, but don't hesitate to ask. After all, a burnt-out and crabby husband does not a good caregiver make. And believe me, there will be times when you are burnt out and crabby. "Even the best caretaker gets fed up occasionally," says Carol Shields, a Canadian novelist who was diagnosed with stage III breast cancer. "I recognize when that kind of care-taking exhaustion happens—when I've just asked for too many things all on top of each other, things I don't really need done at that moment. I try to back off."

I hope your wife is as understanding. And I hope you won't feel guilty asking for a little time off. "I couldn't have gotten through it if I wasn't able to have some space," says Gary Krimstein, 40, of North Potomac, Maryland. Even if it was just time to watch a movie or go for a bike ride. "I think Becky respected that."

David Moyer, 52, was looking forward to his annual fall hunting trip, but when his wife Brenda was diagnosed with cancer, he figured he'd have to skip the excursion. "I just said, 'Is it okay if I go?'" and Brenda, 52, said, "Sure." Her daughter filled in at home, and David got to be captain of the deer-hunting camp for 3 days. Back in Macungie, Pennsylvania, David even figured out a way to spend time working in his woodshed while Brenda was recuperating from chemo treatments. He worried that if he wasn't in the house, she might need him, and then what? The solution: walkie-talkies. And they weren't just in case of an emergency. "We talked dirty to each other," David confides with a chuckle.

Social worker Frank McCaffrey recalls a husband who would go for his "Route 128 therapy"—long solo drives on a New England highway listening to his favorite music. "That was very soothing to him." It could be a time to think things through—or to empty out your mind and think about nothing.

Other husbands find pleasure in material objects, and there's nothing wrong with that. Jeffrey Berger had been thinking about buying a Saab convertible for years. His wife, Diane, said, "This is going to be a hard year for us and who knows what will happen? Why don't you just get the Saab and enjoy it now? You can use it to drive me to chemo." But she wasn't completely thrilled by the prospect. Diane felt less than sexy with her bald head. And Jeffrey would look extremely cool in his Saab convertible. His solution: vanity tags that said ILVDIAN. "My heart is on my license plate," he jokes. As Diane went through the treatments, he says, "We tried to treat ourselves well and have fun." And they did—even when her wig almost blew off on a drive with the top down.

Exercise can be a balm, too. "I was pretty fanatical about fitness," says Frank Sadowski, who lives in Seattle, where he's vice president for consumer electronics merchandising at amazon.com. He loves to bike, but damp Seattle winters don't offer the best conditions for cycling. "I started spinning three times a week, like a religion," he says. "I was going to the gym almost every day, for at least 45 minutes to an hour, on the way home from work. I was pretty fanatical about not dissipating myself."

"I tried to exercise," says Colton Young, "because breast cancer is a marathon, a physical marathon." Friends would ask how he felt, and he'd say, "like a wolf, a lone wolf running across a frozen lake, covering mile after mile after mile, regardless of terrain, physical condition, level of hunger, just moving, continually moving, and making it look somewhat easy."

When friends would call journalist Steve Roberts and ask what they could do to help during his wife Cokie's treatments for breast cancer, he'd say, "Play tennis." With him, that is.

Earl Medansky continued his pushups and weightlifting while his wife, Cookie, was going through her treatments. The Chicago lawyer didn't work as late as he usually did, but he still made time to stop at the gym on the way home. And that was okay with Cookie. "You cannot live your life around someone else," she believes.

Sometimes a friend would say to her, "He's working out?"—as if that were a sign of Earl's callousness.

Cookie would calmly reply, "He makes himself strong so he'll be strong for me."

even though guys think they're expert fixers, they may just glaze over when confronted with a real-life dilemma. One technique is to think about how the stupidest person you know might handle the problem, suggests Matthew Loscalzo. You'll then come up with a stupid solution—which actually could lead to a useful thought about how to help.

To make matters more complicated, as the months of treatment go by, your job as caregiver will change. In fact, it could change from day to day, because one day your wife might want you to cheer her up, and the next day she might want you to commiserate with her. (For more on how best to handle the very delicate matter of your wife's feelings, see the next chapter, beginning on page 48.)

YOUR DAILY CHORES

All that said, there is one rule that seems to apply to all breast cancer husbands: Helping around the house is a very good thing. Your wife will be busy coping with cancer treatments. So she will almost certainly not have the time or energy to attend to tasks she may normally do around the house. And while love may keep you together, it sure won't clear the table or do the laundry.

Another rule for the home front: No matter how hard you try, you'll inevitably do something wrong. "I'm a guy, I'm gonna break stuff, I know my soup's not going to be that great," says Dave Como, 35, of Pittsburgh. Maybe you'll load the dishwasher incorrectly. You'll fold the clothes sloppily. You'll commit the cardinal sin of vacuuming from north to south instead of east to west. (Or is it the other way around?) Oh, and by the way, this is not the time to rearrange the kitchen in any way, shape, or form.

Whatever you volunteer to do, honor your commitments. Cathy Kautz, 51, and her husband, Tom, 52, still joke about her first day home from the hospital after her mastectomy 6 years ago. She wanted to take a bath and wash her hair. Tom told her, "I'll help." But first he wanted to work on the sprinkler system in their Parkland, Florida, yard. "I'll be right back," he said.

Hours later, Cathy gathered up her drains and bathed herself. When Tom finally came in, he was puzzled: "Why didn't you wait for me?" Cathy said, "I couldn't wait all day." (Although she understood that he just needed to do a little physical labor to cope.)

Some men think they can do it all, from sprinklers to shampoos. They may even resent family or friends who take over chores. "It's a guy thing," says Colton Young. "At first I didn't want any help. 'Everybody stay away. I can handle all of this. I can manage all this. I can work, I can travel for work, I can manage the family.'" He could do the laundry, do the dishes, take care of the kids, hold down his job, and care for his wife as well. "Sleep—who needs sleep? Four hours, that's enough."

It wasn't. "Swallow your pride," Colton advises other breast cancer husbands, "and take what's offered to you." His neighbors watched the couple's two kids, brought over food, even hired someone to come and clean their house. Colton learned that he couldn't do it alone.

"After it was all over," he says, "we threw a massive party, invited all those people that helped us, and had a keg of beer and all the food they could eat. We thanked 'em all day long." If any of those friends and neighbors ever needs any help, Colton knows that he and Kathleen will be glad to pitch in.

What if no one's offering a hand? Don't be shy about asking. If your wife drives carpool and can't handle her share, see if the other carpool drivers might pitch in. If offers of assistance are vague, make sure you give specific ideas. When someone wants to help, tell them they can make dinner—and let them know if your family hates tuna noodle casserole.

Conversely, the parade of helpers might seem overwhelming. "It's possible that because so many other people are helping, the husband just stands back and doesn't even offer to help," observes Dr. Weiss, the oncologist. The wife might be resentful—why isn't he doing more? The husband might be resentful, too. Friends are flocking to the house, talking to his wife, calling on the phone to arrange assistance. He might feel they're intruding.

In that case, tell your wife, "It's great that you have all this help, but you're not asking *me* to help you."

WHAT WOMEN DON'T WANT

Some men think they have to be "über-husbands" to be good caregivers. "Some guys go into overdrive. They take on everything to make it as easy as possible," says Frank McCaffrey, a clinical social worker who counsels breast cancer husbands at Beth Israel Deaconess Medical Center in Boston. "The risk is that some women still want to do what they can do. They don't want to be told to sit down and rest. They feel less meaningful. They lose their sense of identity and self-esteem." Psychologist Beth Meyerowitz, Ph.D., a professor of psychology and preventive medicine at the University of Southern California who does research on cancer survivors and their partners, agrees. "People don't like solicitous overconcern. If you can be supportive and helpful without making the person feel dependent, that seems to be the most helpful kind of support."

For further details, just ask the ladies of the Lunch Bunch.

The Lunch Bunch is a cancer klatch in the Washington, D.C., area: a group of women who have fought (and, in some cases, are still fighting) breast or ovarian cancer. Each week, they gather for a noonday repast, and for honest talk about what it's like to live with cancer. I had the privilege of dining with them on a chilly Friday in February.

Over soup and salad, the women told me how much sympathy they feel for the poor, neglected breast cancer husband. One woman says, "When I hear of somebody getting a diagnosis, I always send a card to the support person." She'll write: "You need some support. I'm here to support you." So, yes, women really do care about us poor guys. Then it was time for the main course: The Things Caregivers Do Wrong.

"I had a very supportive husband, but it drove me crazy," says a woman with a no-nonsense demeanor. Let's call her Betty. Mr. Betty had just retired. He'd been busy for 35 years in the workplace, and now he was going to get busy at home, taking care of his wife. He offered to be the chef—and that was fine—but he didn't know what he was in for. During chemotherapy, Betty's mouth sores made her one tough customer to cook for. One week, she craved salty soup. The next week, it burned her increasingly tender gums. Her poor husband would feel bewildered, rejected. Gee, last time she loved this food. What's the deal? She's rejecting my cooking!

Betty, meanwhile, didn't want to hurt his feelings. "It's hard on the wife to say, 'Please, don't sauté onions for the next 4 months because the smell makes me sick!'" Betty says. A moment of tension over soup or onions seems so fixable, but neither one of them could talk about it then, and Betty says, "We still haven't talked about it years later." Her advice to overly sensitive husbands: "Go with the flow."

A tall, good-natured woman in her 40s—let's call her Viv—had a house-husband at her beck and call. She was diagnosed in the month of November. Her husband's employer told him to go home until the first of the year at full salary. Now that's an enlightened employer.

Two and a half weeks later, Viv sent him back to work.

"I couldn't take it anymore," she says. "He was driving me crazy, trying to find things to do that didn't need to be done."

Another wife chimes in, "There's only so much you can take of a husband."

And Viv says, "There wasn't a whole lot for him to do. I wasn't an invalid. I could go get a drink of water."

A suggestion bubbles up from the crowd. "That's when you teach him how to wallpaper. Or send him to a friend's house and say 'Paint her bathroom.'"

"My doctor said: 'Stay out of crowds,'" Viv continues. "My husband knew I was going to keep going to the store." So he analyzed traffic patterns at the local supermarket and decided that Wednesday afternoon was the time when the crowds would be the least madding. Of course, weekends were out of the question. "So maybe I should go at 3:00 A.M.!" Viv says with a laugh. Shoppers Food Warehouse was also on the forbidden list, because he didn't want her to bag her own groceries.

That's why her husband was back at work before he knew it.

Sal would have liked to send her husband back to the office, too, except he had retired. She was working and he was king of the home front when she was diagnosed. "And suddenly, I'm at home," says Sal. She didn't have her friends at work to give her support. And her husband was determined to treat her like a queen.

She'd get up to do something. "He kept saying, 'No, I'll do that, I'll do that.' What am I gonna do? I felt like I had died and life had passed me by. I said, 'I'll go to the grocery store.' He'd say, 'What do you want?'"

"I wanted to go to the grocery store is what I wanted."

There she was stuck at home with a totalitarian caregiver. She had nothing to do except watch television. It was the summer of the O.J. Simpson trial, and that became her life. "I watched the trial from beginning to end. It was someplace for me to be.

"He wanted to be there for me," she recalls ruefully. But he made her feel like "the interloper at home."

As my meal with the Lunch Bunch drew to a close, one message became very clear: Your wife is the boss. You, the caregiver, should serve at her pleasure. Take your cues from her as to which tasks she wants you to do around the house—and which ones she needs to continue doing herself.

A BUMPY ROAD

By now, you probably realize that no matter how stellar a caregiver you are, things may not always go smoothly.

"When both people in a relationship are well, things work in synchronization," says McCaffrey. "But the more stress, the more everybody is worried. Either spouse can be distracted and not right on top of the other person's needs. I tell husbands that it's not unusual for the woman to turn inward. She's more focused on herself, and what it's going to take to get through these tests and treatments. She's less aware of the other person. That's not true of every relationship. In some, the wife is still able to play a caring role."

But it's inevitable that she won't be as tuned in to your feelings as she might usually be. "I know many couples that argue and bitch all the time," says breast cancer husband Frank Sadowski. "We don't do that. We're very respectful in the way we deal with each other." But when his wife, Laura, was going through chemo, and he was trying his best to be a good househusband, he sometimes felt a little unappreciated. When he cleaned up or put things away, it was never the way she would have done it—that was the message he got from her tone of voice and her body language. "Instead of 'Thanks for busting your ass from 6:00 A.M to 10:00 P.M.,' it was like, 'You mean you didn't mow the lawn today?' I just wanted to go out and scream." Plus, he felt guilty: "God, she's got cancer and I'm pissed off at her? But the fact of the matter was, I was pissed off. And in the great scheme of things, that's a very human reaction—to feel sorry for yourself."

Other husbands have shared similar feelings. Am I really doing a good job? She used to tell me I was, and now she doesn't. The men seem to think that if they ever dared ask for feedback, the earth would stop spinning. "She's angry because she's not feeling supported in the way she wants to feel supported," says psychologist Anne Coscarelli, Ph.D., who directs the UCLA Ted Mann Family Resource Center at the Jonsson Comprehensive Cancer Center. "He feels he's done everything he can do, and if it's not appreciated, he's

---

HUSBANDING HER ENERGY

As his wife's caregiver, Jay Grogan made sure they both had enough energy to cope. "The most precious thing you have is energy," the 44-year-old Dallas lawyer explains in his down-home drawl, "and energy gets zapped by fatigue."

After Lynn's diagnosis 12 years ago at age 34, Jay wanted her to be able to spend her precious reserves the way she wanted to. Some friends consume your energy with their negative feelings, he points out. (You know who they are.) Others give you energy. The couple sought to include the latter in their lives, and didn't feel bad if they excluded the energy sappers.

Jay suggested that Lynn reassess her volunteer work. A stay-at-home mom, she had a heap of school and church responsibilities. "In her mind, it was like, 'I made a commitment,'" he says. "My point was that you made the commitment before you knew you were going to have chemo. It's time to reevaluate. It's not like you're breaching a contract. You're saying, 'I've got changed circumstances.'"

He didn't want Lynn to give up activities that meant a lot to her, but he didn't want her to feel as if she had no choice. It was hard at first, he says. "She was as driven, as Type-A, as anybody." Another lesson to learn: Since people are always offering to help, let them pitch in.

You and your wife have a choice about how to handle phone calls and e-mails, too. "Don't be a captive of that stuff," says Jay. "I mean, it will victimize you." Change your answering machine to say, "We're not able to return all your calls. Please understand—and let us know if it's urgent."

If you don't call back, people will indeed understand. And if they don't, well, that's their problem, not yours.

angry." So each of you retreat from the other at a time when you really need to come together.

That's what Will David* was feeling during the chemo months. "There may be an element of my wife feeling I'm not attentive enough, not asking how she's doing enough. In moments of anger, she says, 'If you're not with me and won't give me the support I need, then this marriage is not worth it to me.' I said, 'You have to tell me what you want. I can't always figure it out. I'm so busy and distracted and anxious, too. I wish you would tell me.' But she feels she shouldn't have to tell me."

The husband may need a bit of support, too, says David Spiegel, M.D., associate chair of the psychiatry department at Stanford University School of Medicine, who has studied the benefits of support groups for breast cancer patients. If a woman tells him that her husband is clueless, he tells her, "If I were your husband, I wouldn't know what you wanted. Can you make it clear to me?"

The woman may be angry that she even needs to ask for help with tasks she once handled routinely. Dr. Spiegel recalls a breast cancer patient, ill with metastatic disease, who was making tacos for her husband and son but didn't have any lettuce in the house. Her husband said, "I'll go buy some lettuce." The wife screamed, "Can't you eat tacos without lettuce?" If he had told her the tacos would be just fine without the lettuce, Dr. Spiegel adds, she probably would have lashed out, "What, can't you go and get some?"

What's the solution? "Give her a hug, reassure her that you love her," Dr. Spiegel advises, "and say, 'Honey, I'm as frustrated as you are. But let's not fight with each other.'"

A session or two with a therapist could help. You and your wife are then in a neutral place where you can each say what you're feeling. If the idea of a therapy session in the middle of chemo seems daunting, then try talking to each other. Not *at* each other, but *to* each other. First, you tell your wife how you're feeling. Then, listen to her tell you how she's feeling. Don't try to "fix" or critique each other's feelings—just listen. If all goes well, empathy will kick in. You'll come to understand how she's feeling, and she'll get a sense of your feelings. And maybe you'll be better communicators in the future.

In the end, you're not merely the new maid. Even if you do a stupendous job as a housecleaner, your wife will crave your support in other ways. "It got to the point in that initial period," says Kathleen McCarthy, remembering the early days after diagnosis, "when I would say to Colton, 'Stop vacuuming the rug. I understand the dishes need to be done. I appreciate what you're doing. But I would rather you sit with me and talk to me.' Here I am watching him go past the door, listening to him do things throughout the house. That wasn't what I wanted from him. And most of the time he catches himself and realizes, 'If I just listen to her and let her say her piece, she'll feel better.'"

And so will he.

TIPS ➢ ➢ ➢

1. At a loss for what to do as a caregiver? Ask your wife for a to-do list.
2. At www.menagainstbreastcancer.org, you'll find caregiver tips and other helpful information aimed at husbands.
3. To relieve caregiver fatigue, take time for stress-busting activities—whether watching sports on TV or going for a 5-mile run. Just make sure your wife doesn't need you before you take off (or zone out).

➢ BONUS TIP

If your wife craves company but isn't up for long visits, volunteer to act as the traffic cop. Carol Shields's husband, Don, would take friends up to her bedroom (along with a pot of tea), then return in an hour and say, "I think it's time."

Your Wife's Feelings

Why it's better to hear than to cheer

Your wife is reeling from her breast cancer diagnosis. She's terrified by the thought of the treatments. She's afraid of making the wrong choices. And she's haunted by the fear that she will not be a breast cancer survivor. One night, as the two of you are getting ready for bed, she begins to tell you how upset . . . and worried . . . and traumatized she is. Your response:

a) Cheer up, honey, the doctor said things aren't that bad.
b) Can we talk about this later?
c) I understand how you're feeling. Is there anything I can do to make you feel better? Or do you just want to talk about it?

I probably don't have to tell you that "c" is the right answer. And I definitely don't have to tell you how hard it is for men to sit back and listen.

RAH, RAH, RAH, SIS BOOM BLECH

Even in the best of marriages and even in the best of health, husbands and wives don't dwell in perfect harmony. We miscommunicate, and we make up, and life goes on.

But when breast cancer comes into the picture, communication becomes more critical than ever. And guys often go terribly wrong in the all-important arena of feelings. Our wives want to tell us how they're feeling; we may feel uncomfortable listening.

Part of the reason may be our male desire to fix things. And how do you fix a bad feeling? By making it go away, of course! By changing the subject, by avoiding the topic, by trying to convince your wife to cheer up. It's as if there's a crack in the wall, says social worker Patricia Spicer, coordinator of the breast cancer program for CancerCare, the national organization, and the solution is to cover it over with wallpaper so no one will know it's there.

Part of the reason may be selfishness. Let's face it, life is more pleasant for a breast cancer husband if his wife is upbeat and optimistic instead of dark and gloomy. But in the end, your wife may learn not to talk to you about how she's really feeling. That just can't be good.

And part of the reason might be that many guys are emotional virgins. Let's say your wife is telling you how bad she feels, and you listen empathetically—you really feel what she's feeling. You might then find yourself feeling vulnerable, threatened, disturbed. Those are tough emotions for anyone to deal with, but women often have had more experience working through such feelings than men have had, explains psychologist Richard Ogden, Ph.D., of Bethesda, Maryland, who lost his wife to breast cancer and now leads the men's breast cancer support group that I attend. He believes that women may also be constitutionally wired to better tolerate deep emotions. (In the immortal words of humorist Dave Barry: "Your wife is—face it—a woman.") As for us guys, even a little wave of emotion can be unsettling. "To use a metaphor," says Dr. Ogden, "you can drown in a bathtub if you don't know how to swim."

Rather than learning to stay afloat in treacherous bathtub waters, many men go into cheerleading mode. I know I did it, and I bet you've done it, too. Cheerleading may spring from genuine altruism. We just don't want to see our wives suffer. And maybe we think that if we're feeling confident about winning the battle with cancer, our wives should share our positive attitude, too. But people cope differently, says Mary Ann McCabe, Ph.D., the licensed clinical psychologist, who counsels families with cancer. "You have to respect that. What works for one person doesn't work for another."

I'm not saying you should *never* be a cheerleader. "Women may want an optimistic person who is going to coach them, help them get information, advocate for them when they're too tired or beaten down or ill from treatment," says Matthew Loscalzo, a social worker and director of patient and family support services at the University of California at San Diego Cancer Center. Bernie Smith, who eventually lost his wife to the disease, remembers how his wife deputized him to be her minister of optimism, to give her hope when others felt there was none.

But breast cancer patients don't necessarily want a round-the-clock pep squad. And a word to the wise: Stay away from sports metaphors. One

---

SHE'S SCARED, I'M NOT

Ted Smith didn't know what to say to his wife, Laurie, when she was gripped by the fear of breast cancer. Diagnosed 7 years ago at age 46, Laurie certainly had reason to be anxious. She had a mammogram that turned up suspicious specks. She drove 35 miles from her home in Conway, Arkansas, to Little Rock for the biopsy. The cells in the tissue sample were malignant. Attempts at lumpectomy were not successful because the cells were too scattered. So the doctors recommended a mastectomy. "It was a further huge kick in the stomach," she says. "You're so bound by great fear and anxiety, trying to make the right decisions about surgeries, trying to do research."

Ted, on the other hand, was optimistic. He was relieved that they'd found the cancer early and that, according to the doctors, the chances it might spread were low. But he felt as if he couldn't share his positive outlook with Laurie. He admits that in times of stress, he tends to clam up, lest he say the wrong thing. And he was sure she wouldn't have wanted to hear what he had to say. "She would have said, 'And your medical degree is from . . . ?' "

Finally, Laurie's doctor spoke up. He told her to put down the books on breast cancer. He told her to stop over-woman recalls how her boyfriend used to trot out a baseball motif to boost her spirits: "This is the ninth inning and there are two outs, but we are going to knock this ball out of the park." The fourth or fifth time she heard it, she was ready to knock *him* out of the park.

JUST LISTEN

You can't go wrong by just listening. "One thing I try to tell guys whose wives are newly diagnosed is that there may be moments when their wives are upset and scared and talking about those feelings," says social worker Frank McCaffrey. "You don't need to rush in and say everything is fine. It's a time to acknowledge what they're feeling. A time to be quiet, to listen, to say something like, 'No matter what happens, you know I'm going to be there,

---

whelming herself with information. She needed to hear that, so she could begin to let go of her fear. Ted was grateful: "He could tell her that and I couldn't. I could see it, but I knew it would be poorly received."

What if Ted had spoken up? Laurie says, "It probably would have offended me. I would have thought he's not as interested in this as I am." Then she reconsiders: "I don't think I would have gotten mad. I think the most important thing is for people not to be afraid to ask questions of each other, and to really share what they're feeling."

Ted agrees: "I'm not a big talker and not a very good listener, but I would tell a husband to talk more and listen more. I spent a lot of time feeling inadequate because I didn't really know what to do. I would tell a husband not to be afraid to talk things out with whomever he needs to, especially his wife."

And how might a husband share his feelings that things aren't as dire as his wife might think? I asked social worker Matthew Loscalzo for a script. He was happy to oblige: "The best thing is to tell the truth: 'Darling, I know you are seeing the situation as very bleak. I do not want to minimize or ignore the fact that you're really scared. But the information I have heard is not bleak. How can you and I work as a team to support each other?' "

holding steady in the storm with you.' That's all you need to do. You don't always have to make it better."

"More often than not, I think women want to be heard, to talk about their experiences, to feel their way through things, and to grieve," says psychologist Anne Coscarelli, Ph.D., whose specialty is cancer. "And men want to fix it, they want to solve the problem."

So if your wife wants to complain, the best thing you can do is to let her. When men listen, says Loscalzo, "their wives feel heard, understood, loved, and very connected." The husband's ability to hear and to understand makes the wife feel less isolated. "It wards off fear of abandonment, the fear of feeling vulnerable and exposed," he says. As long as your wife feels that she has you by her side, she'll feel safer.

To sum up: It's better to hear than to cheer.

That's what Cleveland Shields, Ph.D., found when he invited 33 post-treatment breast cancer couples to take part in two 4-hour talkathons. Dr. Shields, a marriage and family therapist and an associate professor at the University of Rochester, wanted to see how the wives viewed their husbands and vice versa.

The biggest complaint from the men was that their wives were too emotional.

One fellow told how his wife would talk about her fears, and he'd tell her, "You only have a 3 percent chance of recurrence, so it's fine, you don't have anything to worry about."

"Everything would be fine if she didn't get so emotional," another husband griped.

Quoting survival statistics was a popular response to a wifely emotional outburst. (Did I mention that there were a number of engineers among the men?)

The wives, on the other hand, wanted their husbands to pay attention to their feelings, to acknowledge and to validate their emotions. In other words: to shut up and listen.

Dr. Shields's golden rule: "Never try to talk somebody out of her emotions."

"The biggest mistake that anybody can make is to minimize emotional pain," agrees Roz Kleban, a social worker at New York City's Memorial Sloan-Kettering. Telling your wife, "Don't be silly, you'll be fine" doesn't make her feel better. Instead, try this: "The doctor said this was going to be okay, and I've got my fingers crossed that he's right; but I sure understand how you can be as worried as you are."

"The motto that I tell guys is, 'Hurry up and do nothing,'" Kleban says. "Sit there, hold her hand. Don't run out and get this, that, and the other thing. Listen to what she has to say. That's the most special thing you can do."

And if she has to cry, let her cry. "I could cry my eyes out with Vern," says Susan Taylor, 51, a breast cancer survivor who lives in Winnipeg. "I didn't want to cry in front of my children, but it was wonderful to do it with Vern. He didn't tell me to smarten up and that it would be okay. And it relieved the pressure greatly. The fear would build up, and the only thing that would relieve it would be to talk about it—and to cry."

In a way, it's like singing the blues. "There is the blues, and that is a sad story set to music," says blues singer and pianist Marcia Ball. "But the blues as a way to exorcise your devils is also a part of that tradition. You don't wallow in your troubles. You talk about them and you exorcise them."

THE POWER OF NEGATIVE WRITING

Medical science endorses singing the blues—or, at least, writing them down. William Goodson, M.D., senior clinical research scientist at the California Pacific Medical Center Research Institute in San Francisco, told me about a recent study from SUNY Stony Brook on Long Island involving patients with arthritis and asthma, conditions that can worsen with stress. Seventy of the patients were told to keep a journal, recording their thoughts and feelings surrounding stressful experiences. Forty-two others were assigned to record their plans for the day.

Dr. Goodson likes to ask people: Who do you think did better—the patients who wrote about past traumas or the folks who focused on their daily plans?

He always gets the same answer: Of course, the people who wrote down their plans would fare better. After all, isn't it an optimistic act to make plans for the future? And shouldn't people who suffer from a chronic disease just "buck up" and get through it with smiles on their faces? The study found just the opposite. Almost half of the writers who looked at past traumas showed improvement in their health—better breathing, less pain. Only about a quarter of the people who recorded their daily plans had any change for the better.

Dr. Goodson, who was chief of the breast clinic at the University of California in San Francisco for 15 years, believes the study has a message for breast cancer patients and their families. "People who say, 'This sucks,' did better in the long run," he says. "If your wife says 'It sucks,' ask her how much it sucks." She's going to feel these bad feelings no matter what. If she talks about them, she'll feel better than if they fester inside. Joshua Smyth, Ph.D., the psychology professor who ran the SUNY Stony Brook study, adds that the patient shouldn't be criticized or stigmatized for expressing negative thoughts. "Then you feel worse."

Annette Stanton, Ph.D., a health psychologist and professor in the UCLA department of psychology, has found similar results in her study of breast cancer patients. Sixty women in the post-treatment phase participated. They all wrote about their experience with cancer, but with different aims. One group engaged in "emotionally expressive" writing—they wrote their deepest and innermost thoughts about their disease. The second group practiced "positive" writing—they recorded any positive changes in their lives that resulted from the breast cancer diagnosis. The third group just wrote down facts about their disease.

Of the three groups, Dr. Stanton found that the emotional writers had fewer medical appointments for "cancer-related morbidities"—that is, fewer visits to the doctor to report fatigue, arm swelling, and other side effects from treatment. They were also less worried about recurrence. Of the other two groups of women, the positive writers had a slight edge over the "just the facts" writers in the morbidity department. Keeping an optimistic journal seemed to benefit women whose natural tendency was to avoid negative cancer-related thoughts. The study doesn't explain why the emotional writers fared the best. Perhaps the women who wrote about their emotions got the worrying out of their system and didn't feel the need to go to the doctor as much for reassurance, Dr. Stanton speculates.

A husband could rush out and buy his wife a journal and tell her what Dr. Stanton has found. But not every woman will be interested in baring her soul on paper. "To propel somebody into expressing thoughts and feelings when they haven't done that before can be threatening and scary," Dr.

Stanton notes. If your wife is not inclined to write, make yourself available to listen. "Sometimes you just have a really bad day with cancer," Dr. Stanton says. "To provide a receptive listening ear, and to sometimes share with your wife that, 'Yeah, this is really awful today,' is useful." Far more useful than the tactic of "protective buffering" that spouses sometimes use, when both partners try to protect each other from negative feelings. "That can leave them both feeling isolated," Dr. Stanton stresses.

If you and your wife are protective bufferers, you might need some lessons in opening up communication. Oncology social worker Patricia Spicer suggests "paired sharing." The two of you schedule half an hour each week during a time when the house is quiet. Have a cup of tea or a glass of wine. And talk. In this exercise, your wife tells you what she's feeling. You repeat it back to her. That means you really have to listen to what your wife is saying instead of figuring out your response to her feelings. Then you tell her your thoughts. And she echoes them. "It's amazing what you hear," Spicer says. And what you don't hear. It's eye-opening to think you're parroting your spouse's feelings, only to have your spouse say, "I never said that."

One of the points of this exercise is to let both partners express their negative feelings. "Your whole life has been turned upside down. How can you not be angry?" asks Spicer. "You need to know that it's okay to have negative feelings; it's okay to be angry; it doesn't make the disease worse."

But keeping those feelings inside might be detrimental to your health. In a study published by the *Journal of Psychosomatic Research* in 2000, psychiatrist Karen Weihs, M.D., of the George Washington University Medical Center, assessed 32 breast cancer patients. These women had had a recurrence of their cancer, and it had spread beyond the breast. Dr. Weihs looked at three points: Did the women report high or low levels of anxiety? Did they keep their emotions "restricted" or let them out? And did they live longer or shorter than predicted, based on the severity of their metastasis?

Patients with high anxiety did not live as long as predicted. But the same was true of patients who didn't express their feelings, regardless of their anxiety level. This small study is a "first step," Dr. Weihs says, but she believes it is an indicator of the potential negative impact of chronic anxiety—and of repressing emotions.

In a related study that has been accepted for publication in *Psychosomatic Medicine*, Dr. Weihs looked at newly diagnosed women undergoing chemotherapy. The women were, of course, distressed. But the patients who accepted their distress as a normal reaction reported that the distress diminished over the next 18 months. And those less-distressed women had a better survival rate. So if your wife has the urge to purge her feelings, and you encourage her to share and tell her it's perfectly natural to be upset, you may be doing more than you could possibly realize.

Of course, there are instances when a husband's ear is not enough. When your wife's emotions overwhelm her on a regular basis, when a debilitating depression lingers weeks after the diagnosis, when she seems ready to toss you out of the house for a typical husbandly screw-up like forgetting to gas up the car, when her feelings of helplessness evolve into feelings of worthlessness, when she is cutting herself off from family and friends, that may be a time to suggest that she seek help. A therapist who has worked with breast cancer patients (and couples) might be able to help with talk therapy; your wife can ask a local breast center or her cancer docs for a recommendation. A psychiatrist can do a full evaluation and determine if medication, as well as psychotherapy, might be needed.

But therapists stress that a husband can only make the suggestion. The wife has to be ready, in her own mind, to go forward. And Fran Jenkins* was. "I was in the middle of going through chemo," she recalls, "and the oncologist says, 'Are you depressed?' I say, 'No, I'm fine.'"

Her husband is sitting next to her nodding: Boy, is she ever depressed.

"You don't always know what you're exhibiting to other people," Fran says in retrospect. "I wasn't talking to anybody. I didn't want to talk on the phone. I was over-the-edge depressed." And she's over-the-top grateful that her husband spoke up.

THE BEST MEDICINE

Let's review.

Cheerleading: may be okay occasionally, but only if and when your wife seems to like it, and only if you can do it without negating your wife's feelings.

GUY TALK

"I held Sherry and reassured her. The phrases I said really sound meaningless, but they were heartfelt and I believed them: 'Everything is going to be all right. We will work through this. We'll be strong.' I used a lot of 'we' because we are very dedicated to each other. It wasn't a lot of 'I' and it wasn't a lot of 'you.' It was a lot of 'we.'"

—JEFF DAVIS, 51
Lynnwood, Washington

Listening: very, very, very good.

Therapy: something to bring up if your wife shows consistent signs of significant depression.

And what about jesting?

Sharon Manne, Ph.D., a psychologist who directs the psycho-oncology program at the Fox Chase Cancer Center in Philadelphia, looked at how 150 breast cancer couples used humor as a coping mechanism. In general, "lightening it up a bit" was a positive step, she found. Joking around reduced the woman's distress. Although as you might expect, it depends on the nature of the joke.

A husband must develop a keen sense of what will fly and what won't in the realm of breast cancer. Because you're working a very tough room. All I can say is, let your wife's reaction be your guide. She may feel too sensitive to enjoy a jibe that makes fun of her. One woman said to me, "My husband joked easily but never joked about anything personal. I was very appreciative of that. I know a family where the husband made jokes about his bald wife looking like a monk. That would have been crossing the line for me, saying I looked like a monk."

But some husbands told their wives they looked worse than that—and the wives loved it. Phil Gay told his wife, Carol Stevenson, that whenever he beheld her bald head and sunken eyes, he had the urge to go bowling. He swore she loved the joke. I really thought that Carol must have been a little put off by his teasing. But no, she told me that the bowling joke tickled her funny bone. "We used to laugh a lot, it's just so outrageous," she says.

Brenda Moyer's husband, David, kept her in stitches with corny, but good-natured, jabs. "After 32 years of marriage, we're pretty open with anything we say," David says. "She knows I will always speak my mind. That's the way I go through life." When Brenda opted for a mastectomy to remove the 3-centimeter tumor in her left breast, David teased her that "the other one was always my favorite anyway." Then he called her "boobless in Macungie"—that's the Pennsylvania town where they live. And a "padiddle"—the nickname for a car with only one headlight working. When she went to purchase a prosthesis, he said, "Yeah, we're going for her tit fit today."

Did she mind all those jokes? "No," Brenda says without a moment's hesitation. "He does it in a loving way. And it's the greatest thing in the world to be able to laugh."

"If you don't keep your sense of humor," says David, who's been teasing his wife for 32 years, "cancer will worry you to death."

THE NEXT BEST MEDICINE

Neither the gift of laughter nor a material gift can vanquish cancer or make up for a lost breast. But a thoughtful present might make your wife feel better, as long as you avoid electric blankets, vacuum cleaners, and kitchen appliances.

"It doesn't have to be something expensive," says Neal Engledow. "If you see a new paperback by an author she likes, buy it and bring it home. I bought my wife a Gameboy before surgery. She's into that stuff. It lets her know you're thinking about her."

But don't overdo it. Especially if you're the kind of guy who never gives gifts. Philadelphia breast radiation oncologist Marisa Weiss, M.D., has seen some of her breast cancer patients unnerved by a shower of presents from a previously inattentive husband. "They had less than a wonderful marriage, problems in their marriage," she says. "Maybe the men weren't devoted before, or there may have been infidelity, or things weren't going great. And when it comes to treatment, they're all over their wives. I'm not sure what it's about—maybe they're feeling guilty about their misbehavior or their lack of attentiveness." And the wives might think, "If he's all over me now, I must be dying."

You know that slightly annoying birthday party cliché—"the best present is your presence." Maybe you should have it tattooed on your forearm.

Meanwhile, all husbands, regardless of their track record, can benefit by hewing to another hoary motto: "Say it with flowers."

Let me explain.

I was the point person for phone calls from doctors, since my wife is a teacher and is hard to reach in the classroom and during after-school meetings. A few days after Marsha's surgical biopsy, the doctor called to report the findings. Yes, the lump was cancerous. Tumor size: 2.7 centimeters. Margins: not clear. We had been hoping for 2 centimeters or less. And there I was, sitting at work at 4:00 P.M. with this unfortunate news and with no way to reach my wife until I walked in the front door at 6:30.

A dear friend called. I told her what the doctor had said. She said, "Get her flowers."

That didn't make any sense to me. How could flowers make Marsha feel better about the size of her tumor and the prospect of more surgery, followed almost certainly by chemotherapy?

Nonetheless, I obeyed orders. I walked to the flower shop around the corner from my office and splurged on a gorgeous bouquet of poppies—Marsha's favorite flower.

I came home, told her the doctor's findings, and gave her the flowers. She hated the news. She loved the poppies.

This whole exchange was somewhat puzzling to me. How could flowers be such a powerful force for good at a time of sorrow? Many months later, I had my floral epiphany. I told a female colleague at work the story of the biopsy report and the poppies, and she said with a sigh, "Flowers, how romantic!"

And then, at last, I got it. Flowers hark back to the days when you were courting your wife, when romance was in the air and breast cancer wasn't. Those pretty petals conjure up carefree days of the past. They're a promise that your love hasn't disappeared. So guys, let me reiterate: You can't go wrong with flowers.

I shared that piece of advice with a breast cancer husband who was falling down on the job. His wife complained to me that he never asked how she was feeling, which made her feel lost and alone. "I'm not expecting him to find a magic wand and wave it," she said. "Asking me how I'm doin'—that would be nice."

"I guess maybe I should have a little more understanding rather than just going on and assuming everything's okay," the husband sheepishly told me. But he's been feeling overburdened himself. His wife quit her job shortly before her diagnosis, so he's been working long shifts. And now, when he comes home, he has to take care of the house because his wife is dealing with her cancer.

So I thought maybe I could fix things. I said to him, "I'll tell you what a friend told me: Get her flowers. Works every time."

Turns out that he and his wife had been in a supermarket a few days before, and she had asked him to buy her a bouquet. "I sort of blew it off," he told me. "In a food store, of all places, you don't get flowers!"

There you have it: definitive proof of the utter cluelessness of men.

So I told him, "Yes. Even supermarket flowers will do."

TIPS ➢ ➢ ➢

1. Empathize, don't criticize.
2. Your wife might want to tell you the same story more than once. It's therapeutic for her—and it's goodhearted of you to listen with a sympathetic ear.
3. If your wife is open to the idea, encourage her to keep a journal and record her true feelings about her cancer. Studies show that women who express their emotions tend to cope better.

➢ BONUS TIP

Looking for some uninterrupted time to talk? Get in the car and go for a leisurely ride in the country.

Your Feelings

You know you've got 'em, but should you share or conceal?

"I asked him to tell me how he felt," recalls Katherine Kim, 72, of her husband, Tye. She had just learned that she had breast cancer, and she wanted to know what was going on in Tye's mind. "He never said anything. You know Asian men—they are so macho."

Occidental males are just as guilty. "Men seem to think if they really let their emotions out, their penises will fall off," jokes therapist Cleveland Shields, Ph.D. "I've never seen it happen yet."

Hey, it's not entirely our fault! Society has conditioned men not to let feelings overwhelm them. In the face of danger, men act, they don't interact, explains therapist Ronnie Kaye, a breast cancer survivor and author of *Spinning Straw into Gold: Your Emotional Recovery from Breast Cancer*. Eons ago, when a wild-eyed woolly mammoth was pursuing a band of manly hunters, the fellows probably didn't pause to share their innermost thoughts about the fact that the behemoth might stomp them to death.

But just because a guy may not be a big talker, that doesn't mean he has a heart of stone. A breast cancer husband is surely experiencing any number of feelings—fear, sorrow, optimism, pessimism, numbness, annoyance at his wife for being too demanding or not demanding enough. And the question is, what do you do with those feelings?

There is no right or wrong answer. I guess I don't have to tell you that men are generally not comfortable expressing their emotions. And even if a husband is willing to speak up, a newly diagnosed woman may not be able to bear hearing how frightened her spouse is. Yet if you do find yourself turning into Mr. Sensitive Guy, and your wife is receptive, sharing your feelings could bring the two of you closer together.

Ultimately, *you* need to decide how much to share, and when to share it. You will, no doubt, make mistakes. At times, you and your wife may feel frustrated with each other. The challenge, psychologists say, is to support your wife with love and companionship whether you are disclosing your feelings or keeping them inside.

THE STRONG, SILENT TYPE

A decade ago, when Katherine Kim got the news, her husband Tye tried to wipe the worried look off his face. And he tried to reassure his wife. "My behavior was as if nothing had happened," says the 73-year-old, who lives in Jenison, Michigan, "and you would be okay, and that sort of thing." He thought that if he were to share his worries, that would only make Katherine worry more.

That's a fairly typical breast cancer husband's response to his own uneasy feelings: suck them up, hold them in, and be strong.

I asked the women of the Lunch Bunch (remember them from the caregiving chapter?) if they'd have wanted their spouses to share their fears. They responded with a resounding roar: "No." They wanted to draw comfort and courage from a strong, solid, and fearless husband.

They didn't want to have to hold his hand and tell him everything was going to be all right.

They wanted him to, in their words, "fake it" if he had to. Ah, the irony.

"Really?" I asked.

"Hell, yes!"

Were they just kidding around?

Hell, no.

A breast cancer husband needs to have a sense of what his wife can tolerate, and when she can tolerate it.

When it comes to expressing your feelings, "I think it totally depends," says psychologist Venus Masselam, Ph.D., who has counseled breast cancer patients in her Bethesda, Maryland, practice. The man's uncensored, dark emotions might be more than the wife can handle in the early days after diagnosis. "It's almost as though it's a kindness," says Dr. Masselam of the masking of a man's fear. "I'm not suggesting that men should never disclose. And I think you have to play it by ear. If a man has to say it, he has to say it. I'm not suggesting that he shouldn't. But it's almost as though by withholding his feelings initially, he's giving his wife the space to have her own feelings."

If everyone is going around saying how scared they are, Dr. Masselam adds, "I don't know where one does muster a sense of hope."

Those words ring true to David Freeman, 40. When he thinks of the tense days after his wife, Yosepha, was diagnosed with breast cancer, he's reminded of a rock climbing expedition with a friend. Scaling a 1,000-foot rock in Colorado, the two of them spied lightning headed their way. "We were screwed," Freeman says. "We knew that if one of us lost it, the other one would, too." So neither climber said how scared he was. They made it down from the rock. They beat the thunderbolts. And then each said to the other, "I thought you were going to lose it."

Yosepha, meanwhile, was grateful for David's seeming fortitude during the cancer ordeal: "She would tell me how my strength helped her." And he didn't tell her that maybe he wasn't as strong as he seemed to be.

Besides, if you do tell your wife you're on the verge of losing it, she may feel she needs to take care of an emotionally wounded husband, which is the last thing she needs to be doing. When breast cancer strikes, the patient needs to take care of herself.

"My husband traveled back and forth to the hospital, lived with his mother-in-law [who'd moved in for the duration], cared for our daughter, and was working in tech sales," recalls Carole O'Toole, 48, of Kensington, Maryland. "I remember thinking this poor man is just going to collapse from the weight of this. But there was nothing I could do about it. I needed him to be strong. And I couldn't have been there for him."

"It's sort of like, 'This is my turn. I need you to be there for me,'" explains Dr. Masselam. "I wouldn't tell anyone not to say how they're feeling; but I think that just as time helps, timing also helps." As time goes by, your wife may be better able to cope with the disease—and with your honest feelings.

And as time goes by, your fears may subside. When my wife was diagnosed with one breast cancer tumor, and then another, and then when doctors found evidence of lymphoma as well, I was petrified. Marsha's surgeon said, "You guys just can't catch a break," which is not what you want to hear from your wife's surgeon. The lymphoma turned out to be a false read, and the doctors seemed optimistic about treatment despite the bilateral cancers. As the weeks went by, I grew less anxious and more confident.

For many couples, those early weeks are a blur of bad news and confusing treatment options—the absolute nadir. Some psychologists say the feeling is as if a terrorist has invaded your happy home. Then you and your wife get used to the news and she settles on a treatment plan, and somehow you feel as if you've recaptured a little of the stability and calm that flew away the minute the word "cancer" first came out of the doctor's mouth. A month after Marsha was diagnosed, we both felt less afraid and more capable of coping.

Many months later, when treatment was done, I asked Marsha how she would have reacted if I had told her how frightened I was early on (and let me tell you, I was plenty frightened). She said, "I would have probably thought you knew something that I didn't know."

TEAM PLAYER

Even a man who is accustomed to sharing his feelings with his wife may feel compelled to button up. Consider the story of Leonard Thomas. Eleven years ago, his beloved wife, Toya, was diagnosed with breast cancer a few months past her 40th birthday. She'd found a lump while doing her monthly breast self-exam and went in for a core needle biopsy. Two days later the doctor

GUY TALK

"Rena's tendency is to think more negatively than I do. So I may have been anxious, but I know my wife well enough to know this is a person I'm not going to share my real anxiety with. It's not going to benefit her."

—PERRY HOROWITZ, 57
Los Angeles

called her at home. "Are you alone or is Leonard there?" the doc asked. "That's when he told us that we had breast cancer," Toya says.

I ask her why she says "we" when she was the patient.

She replied, "Because *we* had breast cancer. We share everything." This is a couple known as "Team Thomas." When I talked to Leonard, he sounded like a teenager in love: "She's jazzercise slim, a former part-time model, a good-looking babe."

The Thomases had already been through one medical nightmare back in 1984, when Toya learned she had a 14-pound benign tumor on her liver and underwent a 6-hour surgery to remove it, followed by a 6-month recuperation.

And here they were again, facing the unknown. The two of them sat up all night after that shattering phone call, cuddled together in a big, wide chair in their bedroom. They sat in the chair and held each other and cried. They were as close as two people could be. Except for one thing.

Leonard didn't divulge his deepest feelings.

Instead, he kept them inside. When the doctor hung up, Leonard's mind ran through a million thoughts. "All I'm thinking is, I'm going to be a widower; my best friend's gonna die; I'm going to have to go through this whole dating thing again. All these selfish things. Every selfish thing you can think of, I'm thinking."

He was also thinking how frightened he was. And he didn't let that out either. "I didn't let anyone know how scared I was," he says. "I wasn't going to let her know. I thought it would have been selfish to tell her how scared I had been when she was trying to deal with this disease."

He finally let some of those feelings out 18 months after Toya's diagnosis, when he went to a training session for a telephone help line for cancer patients. "I just opened up and talked about how I was scared. It was terrific. I wish I had somebody I could have talked to 1½ years before."

Like the Lunch Bunch ladies, Toya wasn't so sure at first that she would have wanted to hear him confess his inner fears. "If he had told me how frightened he was, I would have told him how frightened I was, and we would have wallowed in self-pity."

Leonard says, "But it could have been good." Good to let it all out.

And Toya thinks he might be right. "It could have been good. A relief." And it wouldn't have been a complete shock. Our wives know what we're feeling even if we don't tell them. "I knew he was scared," Toya admits.

None of this surprises Matthew Loscalzo, a social worker and the director of family support services at the University of San Diego Cancer Center. It's a classic case of men are from Mars, women are from Venus. "I have spoken with women whose husbands were dying," he relates, "and they are very comfortable thinking, 'Who's going to help me take care of the children, and how will I pay the bills?'"

Men, on the other hand, feel guilty having such thoughts. They're ashamed. They've been told they shouldn't have any needs; they should protect their families; they should be the warriors. Only they can't protect their wives from the ravages of breast cancer or the treatments. So what else can they do but keep their feelings inside?

CAR CRIERS

Actually, sometimes we confound the experts and let our feelings out.

There are guys who cry right in front of their wives. Bob Sutton, 56, of Damariscotta, Maine, fielded the call from the radiologist with the news about his wife's needle biopsy results. Like my wife, his wife, Marcia, known to all as "Mash," is a teacher and is hard to reach by phone during the day, so he's the designated phone call recipient. The news was cancer and, "I cried like a baby," says Bob. "I just broke out crying in the house by myself. And when my wife got home, I had to tell her. And we both cried together."

And some guys cry when no one's looking.

It happened to me shortly after my wife's diagnosis. It was also shortly after September 11, 2001. On just about every level, I felt as if I had entered a new and horrific era. I remember driving home from an errand on a sunny Sunday, the same sort of blue-sky, no-humidity day that the hijackers struck. Ray Charles came on the radio singing, of all things, "America the Beautiful." His churchy, catch-in-the-throat rendition. I just lost it and tears began falling from my eyes, and I was making these noises that I didn't recognize at first. And then I realized that I was sobbing.

I thought I was going nuts. I was crying in the car listening to Ray Charles sing about "fruited plain"?

But as I talked to other men in the course of researching this book, I found that I wasn't the only car crier. In fact, the car is a sanctuary of sorts for the breast cancer husband. Matt Wey, 45, of Grand Rapids, Michigan, remembers sitting in his car in the hospital garage after spending the day in the hospital while his wife, Jennifer, 39, underwent a mastectomy and reconstructive surgery. "I stayed until they threw me out at about 10 o'clock," he says. "I got to the car, started the car, put my head on the steering wheel, and bawled like a baby. It was the only time it happened." He remembers the welcome sense of relief and release.

"I don't feel like I can cry at home," says Bob Heil, 39, a sprinkler fitter from Wausau, Wisconsin. "It's hard because you've always got to be the rock, you know."

Bob's wife, Brenda, was diagnosed with breast cancer at age 24, shortly after they'd married. (At the time, she told him he should leave her and had even picked out a replacement wife, but Bob wouldn't hear of it.) Brenda had a lumpectomy plus radiation. A few years later she had a recurrence in the breast and underwent a mastectomy. When I met Brenda a year and a half ago, she had just been diagnosed with metastatic breast cancer in her bones. Sometimes she breaks down crying, and Bob keeps in the tears. But sometimes, driving to his construction job, or driving home at night and listening to the radio, he confesses, "I just lose it."

He's not sure what triggers his tears. Maybe they'd just had a fight. Yes, that might be it. Maybe he told her that everything is going to be all right and she got mad at him—because having metastatic breast cancer at age 37 means that nothing is all right, really. Anyway, he remembers losing it in the car.

"Did you feel better afterward?" I ask. "Yeah, I did, actually," says Bob. "Maybe the good cry thing isn't a female thing."

Nope, it isn't. And really, a car is a great place to do it. No one can see you cry in a car. Or at least that's how you feel, wrapped in nearly 2 tons of steel and traveling at 40 mph, cloaked in invisibility and wracked with pain.

Randy Harper is another car crier. He's a music producer in Cleveland and a Southern boy at heart, from "a little bitty town called Clarksville, Georgia." His wife, Hilary, is 40 and, like Brenda Heil, has metastatic disease. Randy figures she's got a chronic disease and together they'll fight it. "I have to admit, I'm not a big cry-in-front-of-you kind of person," he says. "Part of it is the way I was brought up. If somebody else is going through an adversity, you be strong with them and be strong for them. But I have my times. I'm not made out of metal. I did bawl my eyes out on the phone with my dad that first night after Hilary was diagnosed. It was almost like a release, and I needed to do that."

And now he lets it all out in the car. Sometimes he has a good yell at the windshield. And sometimes he sheds a few tears. "That's my little 'feel sorry for Randy' time," he laughs. "I kind of get it out of my system."

Gentlemen, start your engines . . . and your tear ducts.

THE DISCLOSURE DILEMMA

Should you tell your wife you've been sobbing in the Saturn?

In theory and in practice, therapists are in favor of "self-disclosing"—a fancy way to say that you should let it all hang out. Philadelphia psychologist Sharon Manne, Ph.D., has a grant from the National Cancer Institute to look at how breast cancer couples cope, and what would help them improve their "quality of life." One thing she's studying is how husbands respond when their wives "expressed sad affect"—you know, they said that cancer really sucked. In her group of 158 couples, the wife "was better off when the husband responded in kind," says Dr. Manne: "If she said, 'This is really upsetting me' or some other personal statement, and he self-disclosed back"—that is, if he said, "It's hard for me, too." The women whose husbands responded with that kind of statement reported lower amounts of stress and fewer symptoms of depression. "Psychology is proving the obvious," Dr. Manne says with a laugh.

Husbands, she found, "really wanted to be able to talk. They felt neglected in terms of being able to express their own emotions."

Furthermore, it's perfectly natural to be afraid. "A man who does some incredible feat, an astronaut or someone like that, he's brave and he has fear," says actor Michael Tucker. "The man of grace admits his fear and faces it and goes forward. The man who says 'I have no fear' is bullshitting, and everybody knows it. I think the last thing a breast cancer patient needs is a bullshitter."

Frank McCaffrey, a social worker at Beth Israel Deaconess Medical Center in Boston, has talked to many couples after the wife had been diagnosed with breast cancer. When he sits with a husband and wife, he'll tell them that the worst thing the husband has imagined, the wife has probably thought of as well. And vice versa. "What I know from almost every patient I work with," he says, "is that every couple that goes through that initial diagnosis of cancer, they all wonder if the patient is going to live or die. It's one of the first things people think about."

The relationship will benefit if you know how she feels and she knows how you feel, he believes. It can be a relief to disclose. Maybe your feelings won't seem quite as overwhelming once you let them out. Sometimes it's even a relief: "Oh, you were thinking that, too."

During her breast cancer treatments, Linda Ellerbee remembers sharing fears and tears with her partner, Rolfe Tessem. "Allowing yourself to be comforted and him allowing himself to be comforted," she says, "that brought us together in some small ways that turned out to be not so small."

THE URGE TO PURGE

Having a confidante would certainly help a husband in the ongoing task of tackling his own feelings. But in many marriages, a husband's confidante is his wife. Men often don't have a clutch of good buddies who sit for hours and talk frankly about life, sex, and death. If a fellow talks to anyone about these heavy topics, it's probably his spouse. "If something else this devastating had happened that didn't involve my wife, she'd be the first one I'd go to for comfort and sympathy," says Neal Engledow, 56, of Centreville, Virginia, whose wife, Ganga, was diagnosed 2 years ago at age 52. "I didn't feel I could do that. I think I was more worried than she was, and I didn't want her to worry more."

That makes the breast cancer diagnosis even more disquieting. In addition to coping with all the medical news and his wife's moods, the husband is coping with the loss of his best friend's ear. Recognizing the problem, journalist Cokie Roberts gave her husband permission to confide in a friend—a fellow he played tennis with once a week. "I said, 'It's okay; you are not going to invade my privacy.'"

Assuming you could find a support group for husbands, perhaps that would offer comfort as well—or would it?

There's a joke in breast cancer world that husbands and boyfriends would love to come to a support group if it never met, and if they never had to say anything when they got there. Ha-ha-ha. Another problem is our supposedly stunted emotional vocabulary. Radiation oncologist Irene Gage, M.D., who practices at Sibley Memorial Hospital in Washington, D.C., knows of another running gag in the cancer world: At breast cancer support groups, the women all ask each other, "How are you feeling?" and at prostate cancer support groups, the men want to know, "What's your PSA?" Because we guys like to measure. And feelings are immeasurable.

But that's not the whole truth. Psychiatrist Mary Jane Massie, M.D., who sees patients at Memorial Sloan-Kettering Cancer Center in New York City, once ran a monthly support group for breast cancer patients. The husbands were invited to one meeting. Or as she put it, "The wives beat the poor men to death and made them come." A male colleague ran the group with her, and he said, "Mary Jane, I just want to remind you that guys are action-oriented, and women are feelings-oriented, so guys will never tell you how they feel."

Dr. Massie's male colleague decided that a good icebreaker would be to ask the husbands what problems they had, and then see if the group could solve them. He started the exercise, giving each husband a chance to state his problem. Then one guy spoke up and said, "I'm a little disappointed. I had hoped we could come here to talk about how we feel."

For Bob Strickland, 51, a couples group has changed his way of thinking about his wife's breast cancer. Karen, 49, was diagnosed in 1984, 6 years before she and Bob married. Bob used to say there was no way he would go to a support group. "I didn't see any benefit in continuing to talk about it and go through it and relive it. My greatest fear is that Karen will have some type of metastatic disease, and my way of dealing with that fear is to stay distant from it."

But then he began to wonder if he had the wrong attitude. In New Hampshire, where he and Karen live, they joined a support group for cancer couples. "It has certainly strengthened our relationship as a couple," he says. "I had been on the outside too long. We can talk about our feelings now. I feel like maybe I truly understand."

Which is true . . . up to a point. I ask Karen if a man can ever truly understand what it's like to face breast cancer.

She doesn't miss a beat: "No."

MEN ONLY

A couples group may not meet all of a breast cancer husband's needs. Roz Kleban, administrative supervisor of social work services at the Memorial Sloan-Kettering Cancer Center in New York City, is a group maven. She runs groups for patients and for couples. She recalls a couples group in which one woman told how her husband would give a speech to buoy her up: "You're gonna be fine, we're going to the best place for treatments." Only she wasn't sure he really meant it. Kleban asked the husband, "Do you mean it?"

Before he could begin to speak, the wife turned her back to him. Clearly, she did not want to hear his answer. The husband, meanwhile, motioned to Kleban with his hands, giving a sign that he wasn't sure how confident he was that everything was going to be okay.

"It would have been devastating for her to hear that," Kleban says. "She knew it and he knew it.

"That's why I don't like couples groups," she adds. "A support group should be a spot where the partner is free to say whatever he wants to say without having to censor himself."

But men aren't exactly breaking down the door to sign up for the few men-only groups around. "I'm very, very, very frustrated by the fact that I can't get more men to come," says Kleban, who has tried to organize such groups. The problem may be as simple as scheduling or as complicated as the fear of opening up.

If you are lucky enough to find such a group, that doesn't mean it will be a snap for you to "self-disclose."

After my wife finished treatment, I joined a small support group for men, run by a psychologist whose wife was a breast cancer patient and then a breast

CANCER CAMP

When Doug Smith's wife, Carol, was diagnosed with breast cancer at age 34, "it was kind of like a bomb went off," he says. "I think I just went numb." And he stayed numb for a long time.

"I guess I'm not the kind of person who's real helpful or real sensitive," says Doug, of Tracy, California, who turned 41 on the day Carol was diagnosed. "It takes a lot for me to get involved." He did the husbandly things—going to doctor's appointments and the like. But Doug was a begrudging companion. "I was tired of the routine," he admits. "After 6 months I started to get somewhat frustrated with Carol's continued fear of death, her worry about the cancer returning."

Carol began therapy. Doug joined her after a couple of sessions, figuring that the therapist needed his help to make Carol feel better. He learned instead "that I was the one with the deep problems. I had built a wall around me protecting me from the world's miseries, but in so doing I sheltered myself from experiencing real life. I began to feel emotions and I didn't like it. I felt anger and frustration."

Carol's solution was a trip to cancer camp—a pine-scented overnight retreat with activities that offer information and insight to cancer survivors and their families. St. Joseph's Regional Cancer Center in Stockton, California, runs the program.

Doug was not a happy camper. "I don't know why I would want to be around a bunch of people with cancer," he explains. "It seemed creepy." He didn't like singing "Comin' Round the Mountain," and he wasn't a fan of the little name badges.

At the campfire, he had to say something about what he was feeling. "I'm a shy person," Doug says. But somehow, he found the courage to let out his feelings. He told how he'd felt he had been banished to the basement when his cancer casualty. "I started thinking about a group for guys whose wives or partners are diagnosed with breast cancer, because I realize that might have been helpful when I was going through it," says Richard Ogden, Ph.D.

The conversation flows freely when the subject is chemo side effects or the radiation routine. In fact, there's such intense interest in the details of treatment that I thought I'd tumbled upon an essential difference between

---

wife got cancer, and he wanted so very much to get back upstairs to the life he had had before. But then he had come to realize that "it's not so bad down here. I felt I was in a better place." His life was, in many ways, more meaningful than it had been before his wife's diagnosis.

The cancer stories he heard around the campfire reinforced those feelings. "Hearing those people talk was like a religious experience. They touched me at a level that's not normal for me to feel, deep in my soul. I felt the way you sometimes feel when you watch a good movie, when you kind of cry or get a lump in your throat."

Instead of avoiding the emotions that have come into his life, Doug has learned to embrace them—and to share them. Nine years after his wife's diagnosis, he has also come to learn that letting out your feelings isn't a cure-all. "Our marriage is probably stronger in the sense that I'm more aware of what's going on," Doug says of their 21 years together.

Yet revealing his feelings has made him more keenly aware of their differences. He and Carol don't always agree on matters of finance. When it comes to spare time, he likes going to his parents' place in the mountains and she doesn't. "I don't think we would get married today knowing what we know about each other," he says. "I don't think it has anything to do with the cancer. There's been so much compromise, good and bad. At some point you wonder, 'How much compromise is really good for both of us?'

"On the other hand, Carol is the person who knows me the best. There's a happiness with her I can have no other place."

And he's forever grateful to her for taking him to cancer camp. The reluctant camper is now a volunteer counselor, helping other husbands find the courage to say what's in their hearts.

men and women in the breast cancer experience. My thesis: The patient mystically moves through the process while the husband is obsessed with knowing what's going to happen next. Then I shared my idea with a breast cancer survivor, who threw back her head and guffawed. "We'd like to know, too," she said. "Who wouldn't want the script to their life?"

So I revised my theory. My new premise: Men are just not that good at sharing their emotions. You know the song: "Wo-o-o, wo-o-o, wo-o-o . . . feelings?" In our support group, it's more like, "Whoa, feelings." Our conversation grows halting when we try to talk about our fear of breast cancer. Not to mention sex. (We haven't brought it up.) And death. (We're not very good with that topic, either.) "My hope is that as group members become more comfortable with each other, topics can be brought up that have more of an emotional tinge," Dr. Ogden says. A realist, he notes, "That may or may not happen."

But at least we're trying.

TIPS ➢ ➢ ➢

1. Gilda's Club is a network of free "cancer support communities" that offer groups and activities for cancer patients and their family members. See www.gildasclub.org for details.
2. Want to talk? Call Y-ME, the breast cancer hotline at (800) 221-2141. The volunteer counselors are all breast cancer survivors or breast cancer husbands.
3. Or call a university breast cancer center. The staff may know of a support group for couples or maybe even for husbands, and will almost certainly have a therapist available if you'd like to schedule a session.

➢ BONUS TIP

Losing it every once in a while is normal. Maybe you had a bad day at work, and the kids are acting out, and, oh yeah, your wife has breast cancer. "But you have to have a little control over how you break down," says Philadelphia breast radiation oncologist Marisa Weiss, M.D. "You don't want to say something you can't take back. It's not the time to tell your wife you don't think you love her."

The Flustered Father

When—and what—to tell your kids

Dads want the world to be perfect for their children. It's not that moms don't. But men, it seems, have a deep-rooted desire to shield their offspring from pain. The gifted reporter and writer Michael Kelly, who died covering the war in Iraq, summed it up beautifully: "Men, as has been frequently noted, have their failings. The urge to make things right is their counterfailing, their allegory to women's urge to nurture. The male urge is, of course, ridiculous. Who can fix the world, even for one child? But its ridiculousness makes it great. In every life, there should be someone who believes that whatever goes wrong must be fixed, and if not fixed, must at least be made to go away."

So when something goes terribly wrong, a man's instincts may go terribly wrong as well. "My husband wanted to keep the kids in the dark and not tell them anything," recalls Aileen Pruitt, 42, a Florida mother of four and a breast cancer survivor. "He wanted to protect them: 'They're kids, they shouldn't be worrying.'"

That kind of stance can put a mom in a terrible bind. Does she heed her husband, or does she go with her gut feeling that the kids need to know?

Aileen convinced her husband, Ken, that concealment is folly. And indeed it is. "I mean, what are you going to hide from them?" asks Randy

Harper, 44, whose wife, Hilary, 40, has metastatic breast cancer. "The fact that Mom's sick or lost her hair? You ain't gonna hide that long."

Even if your wife does not undergo chemotherapy, you still need to open up. The sin of omission could lead children to think things are worse than they are. "They know something's going on and you're not leveling with them," says therapist Venus Masselam, Ph.D., of Bethesda, Maryland. What they imagine might be 10 times worse than the reality. What's more, you're sending them the wrong message: It's okay to lie when something bad happens.

But what *are* you going to tell them? And how? And who will do the telling—you alone, your wife, or the two of you together?

Much will depend on your family's style of communication, and your children's personalities. That said, here is a rule book of sorts to help you talk to the kids. These two dozen rules were passed on to me by social workers and psychologists, and by mothers and fathers who've had to tell their kids that Mommy has breast cancer.

RULE #1: TELL THEM AS SOON AS YOU CAN

Marsha and I kept the cancer a secret for a couple of days. Telling our daughters on the last Friday of summer vacation, with school looming the next Tuesday, seemed inordinately cruel. Yet concealing this piece of news for 3 short days rocked our home. The kids were on edge anyway: Maya was starting 10th grade, Daniela was moving from elementary school to middle school. When they occasionally ticked off my wife with typical teenage behavior, Marsha would practically burst into tears and issue cryptic utterances like, "You can't understand how this is making me feel."

It made them feel as if Momma were a little loony.

"I knew something was up," Maya now says. "But I brushed it off because I was concentrating on school." In the end, I'm glad she and her sister went off to the first day of school without the cancer cloud hanging over them. Marsha and I picked them up from school that day and told them the truth, which made our home life a little easier.

I've spoken to other families who delayed sharing the diagnosis so the kids could enjoy a milestone event, like a birthday party, or who waited until there was something more to tell. A short delay—perhaps a few days, or at most a week or two—could also help you and your wife gain control of your own emotions. Make sure family members and friends are aware that you're keeping the kids in the dark for a spell. And be sure to tell the children before symptoms appear, and before worried faces or whispered conversations make it apparent that something is not right. Above all, don't delay if the only reason is your own discomfort at breaking the news. The longer you put off the inevitable, the more likely that your children might respond with anger or distress: "Why didn't you tell us sooner?" And the harder it will be for them to trust you to be forthcoming in the future.

RULE #2: DON'T LEAVE IT TO MOM

"From my perspective," says social worker and child life specialist Kathleen McCue, "the mother and father should have absolutely equal responsibility for talking to children about Mom's breast cancer." Children want to know who will care for them, who will be there for them, and who will take over Mom's responsibilities if she's not able, says McCue, who is director of children's programs at The Gathering Place in Beachwood, Ohio, an organization that supports and educates cancer patients and their families. Dad should be there to say, "I will." He should hear the kids' initial concerns and should tell them that even if he doesn't know how to, say, put up his daughter's hair for ballet class, Mom will teach him, or a good friend or family member will lend a hand.

In some cases, Mom may not feel she is up to the task of joining Dad in the first cancer conversation. Once Aileen Pruitt convinced Ken that they had to tell the kids, he was the one who took their four children into the boys' bedroom for the cancer talk. Aileen stayed away. "I knew I couldn't be in there because I would start crying, and that would scare them."

"If there's a need for the children to know before Mom feels she can tell them, and if she really feels she will lose it," says McCue, "it's appropriate for Dad to tell them. But when families ask me, I suggest that the ideal, assuming an intact family, is when both Mom and Dad are there."

RULE #3: BREAK IT TO THEM GENTLY

In other words, don't blurt out, "Mom's got cancer." And don't begin with a somber, "Children, we have some bad news." That might alarm them more than necessary. Tell the children you have something to talk about that's really important, suggests Mary Ann McCabe, Ph.D., a licensed clinical psychologist and an associate professor at the George Washington University School of Medicine in Washington, D.C., who has been counseling families with cancer for 15 years. "That affords them a chance to get their defenses ready." If your family has "family meetings," call a session to order and begin by saying, "Maybe you guys have noticed that Mom's been going to the doctor for the last couple of days, or that Mom and I have seemed a little different." The response from your kids will let you know how much they're aware of. Then you can tell them that you're going to talk about what's going on.

RULE #4: USE THE WORD "CANCER"

Parents may think the word itself will scare the kids. Not using it could scare them more. If you tell very young children that Mommy has a boo-boo, the youngsters might worry that if they bump their head, they'll get what Mommy has. If a child already knows the word "cancer" and the parents don't use it, the child will surely hear it from someone else over the months ahead. And you'll have a lot of explaining to do. As for the child who hasn't yet heard the word "cancer," it will simply be the name for Mommy's illness. Nor should you shun the word "breast." Younger kids may giggle or feel self-conscious about using the word themselves, but they should know that that's where the cancer is.

RULE #5: KEEP IT AGE-APPROPRIATE

If your kids are different ages, one child may ask many questions; another may be satisfied with less information. At the very young end of the spectrum, there may not be much you can say beyond that Mommy is sick with cancer.

GUY TALK

"My older boy was 8. I told him that his mother has cancer. And he had two questions. 'Is it contagious?' And 'Is she going to die?' When my son asked me that question, I didn't boohoo, but I was looking for a Kleenex. That was tough. I told him we're going to do everything we can to keep that from happening."

—COLTON YOUNG, 42
Chalfont, Pennsylvania

Preschoolers—roughly ages 2 to 6—can handle a little more information. They'll definitely want to know what's going on around them. But they do tend to have short attention spans, so aim for simple, reassuring words. "They can understand facts, that Mommy is going to the hospital and the doctor," suggests Hester Hill Schnipper, chief of oncology social work at Boston's Beth Israel Deaconess Medical Center and a breast cancer survivor.

You can tell them that Mommy has something wrong; you can perhaps show them in a drawing (or on a doll or even on Mommy) where the problem is. If your wife is going through chemotherapy, you can tell the children that she is taking medicine to make her better. You don't want to say "bad" medicine, or they might never want to take their medicine again. But you can tell them that it's "strong" medicine, and that the doctors haven't been able to make a medicine that only treats the "sick part," so Mommy may throw up or lose her hair. But all those problems will be fixed when she finishes taking the medicine.

"Talk about the facts," Schnipper says. "Let them ask questions." If they ask, "Is Mommy going to live or die?" you can say, "We hope Mom will be fine. This is our plan for treatment. People do die of cancer, but we have our plan and we expect Mom will be okay." Kids can tolerate uncertainty, says Schnipper. They're resilient. They can "go with the flow."

Young kids are also egocentric (actually, who isn't?). In addition to wanting to know how Mommy got cancer, they will most likely ask, "Did I cause it? Is it contagious? Who will take care of me?" Even if they don't ask, they may be thinking these thoughts. Their older siblings in elementary school may have the same worries.

Fortunately, these are easy questions to answer. It's absolutely not their fault. Mommy didn't get cancer because she worked too hard taking care of them, or because she didn't go to the doctor, or because the kids were bad. You can add that the very best cancer doctors in the world don't know exactly what causes breast cancer. But they do know how to fight breast cancer.

And, of course, it's not contagious.

Finally, you can say that Mom will do the best she can to care for them. You'll be there, too, even though you may have to spend some time taking Mom to the doctor and helping her at home. And maybe family and friends will help out, because that's what family and friends do when someone they love is sick.

Older elementary school kids will probably want to know what cancer is. You can tell them that cancer cells are unhealthy cells that grow too much and can spread in the body, keeping healthy cells from doing their job. But doctors have treatments to eliminate those cancer cells.

As for teenagers, their response will be unpredictable because that's the essence of being a teenager. They might seem resentful. At a time when they're asserting independence, cancer suddenly yanks them back into the fold. Or they may seem disinterested. One teenage son listened impassively to the news of Mom's diagnosis, then asked, "Can I go now?" Keep giving them information even if you don't get an immediate response. And since teenagers and the Internet are joined at the fingertips, you should definitely tell your teens to show you any stories about breast cancer they find on the Web. The information could be wildly inappropriate for your wife's case, or just plain wrong.

RULE #6: DON'T MAKE PROMISES YOU CAN'T KEEP

If you tell your children "everything is going to be fine," McCue says, "that's a promise." But as you no doubt know by now, cancer is an unpredictable demon. Even if your wife's treatments go well, there can always be unpleasant surprises—and unfortunate changes in your family routine. Should Christmas be less merry than usual, or your summer vacation be canceled, children may lash back: "You said everything would be fine, and it's not."

You and your wife can tell the children that Mom will go the doctor and do what she needs to do, and you hope that she will get better. And you can honestly say, "We will do everything we can to keep our family life as normal as possible."

RULE #7: BE TRUTHFUL

A seemingly harmless fib might destroy the bond of trust that you need to maintain with your kids. Besides, youngsters usually have a finely tuned, built-in lie detector. When Wei Chin* and his wife, Betsy, faced cancer, she didn't want to tell the couple's 4-year-old daughter. But Betsy had to say something about her impending baldness, so she said she was getting a short haircut because of the hot weather. The child kept asking, why, why, why. "Why did you get your hair cut short, Mommy?" "So we changed our story," Wei says. "We said, 'Mommy's sick, and she's taking a medicine that is supposed to make her better, but it has the side effect of making her hair fall out.'" They added that when she finishes taking the medicine her hair will grow back. The little girl did not ask about her mom's bald head again.

RULE #8: DON'T TELL YOUR CHILDREN MORE THAN THEY NEED TO KNOW

Of course, that raises the question, how much do they need to know?

The answer: enough to know what's going on.

In general, kids want simple answers, not a dissertation. The first discussion of Mom's breast cancer might consist of delivering the news. You don't have to hold a seminar and discuss all the details of surgery, chemo, and radiation. As a treatment approaches, tell your children what to expect. When kids are prepared for what's going to happen, they can cope better. If your wife is having a mastectomy, give them a heads up at least a couple of days before the surgery. Tell them if she'll have to spend the night at the hospital, and explain that when she comes home, she may feel tired and sore and she won't be able to raise her arm. If she is going for chemotherapy, give them your best sense of what will happen:

"The treatment is on Monday, and Mom probably won't feel very good for 3 or 4 days. But then she should begin to feel better." And ask if there's anything else they want to know.

RULE #9: QUASH YOUR INNER CHEERLEADER

You know you've got one (see the chapter Your Wife's Feelings on page 48 in case you've forgotten). Keep him under wraps. Your kids may be angry, frustrated, fearful, or sad when they first hear the news—just as you were. Your job isn't to banish such emotions. A healthy child will be able to express such feelings and then move forward—just as you are now trying to do. Instead of trotting out happy platitudes, tell your children that you know how they're feeling, and they can always come to you to talk. It's an honor to be the go-to guy, and you want to make sure your kids know you'll always have time to listen.

RULE #10: DON'T HOLD IN THE TEARS

"I've heard fathers say they sat with their kids and started to cry," McCue says. To her mind, that's just fine, and far preferable to Dad the Stoic. By showing your children an honest response from your heart and soul, she says, you "give them permission to let out their own feelings."

RULE #11: GIVE CANCER A PUNCH

With Mom busy dealing with cancer docs and treatments, Dad is the one who needs to pay attention to how the children are doing. If your kids are mad at Mom for being sick, they may disobey her wishes, blow up at something trivial, or pick a fight with a sibling. Or they could lash out at you over something trivial, because how could they dare get angry with poor, sick Mommy? Don't take it personally. But do try to take action. "That's a great time for a dad to say, 'You seem really angry,' and to help the kid express that anger," says McCue. And it might be with a punching bag. At The Gathering Place, McCue keeps a sturdy laundry bag filled with Styrofoam peanuts; she invites angry kids to have at it. "Sometimes they might not even understand why they're punching. But they know that hitting something for a while feels better.

"This is something that Mom probably wouldn't do, but dads may be comfortable with that kind of expression," she says. If your kids lash out or melt down, bring out the punching bag: "Say, 'This is how we feel about cancer in our family,' and let 'em go at it." When they're finished, you might want to take a punch or two yourself.

For a child who's not inclined to punch, Dad might try a quieter way to help handle worries. Set a specific time to talk about anything troubling—say, half an hour on a weekend afternoon. Then take a walk together to show that it's time to stop worrying.

RULE #12: KEEP THINGS AS NORMAL AS POSSIBLE

Everyone finds comfort in rituals and routines, even homework. Yes, tell the kids they'll still have to study and practice piano—and that they shouldn't worry about who's going to take them to their soccer games. And if it comes down to dusting and vacuuming versus taking the kids to their Saturday match, I don't have to tell you which to do. Just don't tell your wife where you read that it's okay to let the dust bunnies multiply.

And don't shut your wife out of the kids' lives by being an overprotective breast cancer husband. David Spiegel, M.D., associate chair of psychiatry at the Stanford University School of Medicine, spends a lot of time studying breast cancer families. He recalls a dad who told the kids, "Don't bother Mother with your homework." Mom yelled, "I can't cook dinner, I can't do much, but I can help with homework!"

RULE #13: TRY NOT TO SHIP THEM OUT

When Mom goes to the hospital for surgery, Dad often isn't sure what to do about the kids. Should he set up a sleepover or arrange for them to stay at home? Especially in those tense first weeks, kids may crave their own beds. If you can find a family member or friend to stay with them until you get home, the kids won't feel quite as unsettled.

RULE #14: DESIGNATE A STAND-IN FOR QUESTIONS

There may be times when you and your wife aren't going to be there for the kids. Maybe you'll be caught up in treatment agonies, or just plain too tired. And sometimes the kids will want to talk to an adult who's not you. The solution is to name a pinch hitter, most likely a family member or an especially close friend. Tell the kids they can call that person any time they have questions or thoughts about Mom's breast cancer.

RULE #15: SPREAD THE WORD AT SCHOOL

It's not up to the children to decide whether you tell their teacher and guidance counselor. You *will*, because that's part of your responsibility as a parent—to let the school know what's happening in your kids' lives. Because youngsters want to be just like everyone else, particularly at school, urge the teacher and counselor not to inquire about Mom's health in front of other students (but suggest that private inquiries are perfectly appropriate). Teachers and counselors can also be helpful allies. Ask if they'll let you know of any unusual behavior—moping, failure to do work, distractedness. In turn, your kids might find it comforting to confide in a beloved teacher or counselor.

As for telling your children's friends—that decision is up to the kids. But you should make your children aware that word is out about Mom's breast cancer. They might prefer telling their best friends instead of having those pals learn the news from another source.

RULE #16: SEEK SUPPORT FOR YOUR KIDS

"They may have a powerful sense of being alone, the only one they know who has a parent with cancer," says social worker Jill Taylor-Brown, director of psychosocial oncology and supportive care at CancerCare Manitoba. If there's a cancer center in town, see if the center ever runs support groups for kids. A meeting with a therapist who has tackled this topic might also prove productive. The therapist can speak with the family as a whole, or just with your kids if you have concerns (or if the children have concerns that they're uncomfortable raising with you and your wife).

Reading a book like *Sam's Mommy Has Cancer* might help, although McCue notes that any book is going to be about one family's experience, which is not necessarily your family's experience. Make your own book, she suggests—a helpful tool for kids ages 3 to 8 or 9. It doesn't have to be

---

READING LIST

A number of books help kids cope with a parent's cancer diagnosis. Some give advice to adults on what to say and do; others are meant to be read aloud to youngsters. Kathleen McCue, director of children's programs at The Gathering Place and herself the author of a first-rate guide, *How to Help Children Through a Parent's Serious Illness*, recommends the following titles. The books can be ordered through online bookstores.

When a Parent Has Cancer: A Guide to Caring for Your Children by Wendy Harpham ($26, HarperCollins). The Dallas physician and mother of three was diagnosed with non-Hodgkin's lymphoma in 1990. Her thorough and helpful book, appropriate for families coping with any sort of cancer diagnosis, is packaged with a picture book, *Becky and the Worry Cup*, with quotes from kids recalling what life was like when their parent became a cancer patient.

The Paper Chain by Clare Blake, *et al* ($8.95, Health Press). This picture book for school-age children is simple, sweet, and true to life. When Mom is diagnosed with breast cancer, two young brothers pitch in at home, complain about how boring it is to help out, get into a fight over nothing, and learn that Mom's energy—and hair—do come back when treatment ends.

Moms Don't Get Sick by Pat Brack with Ben Brack (out of print, used copies sold for various prices under $10, Melius Publishing). An excellent resource for parents and children, this 106-page book offers a "she said, he said" account of a mother's battle with breast cancer, with alternating passages from Pat and her son, Ben, who was 10 when she was diagnosed. Together, they offer a candid portrait of a house where cancer has come to live for a spell—no one nags the kids to clean up the bathroom; Ben steals things from his mother's room "partly to get back at Mom for getting sick." And in the end, Ben learns that "families are what it is all about and ours is more than okay."

elaborate: a loose-leaf binder, some paper, and a pen are all you need. You can draw stick figures (or artistic kids may be more ambitious). Let your children help you write the story: Mommy has cancer. She went to the hospital. She is taking medicine that makes her lose her hair. They may want you to read them the "story" from time to time. When they stop asking to hear it, you'll know they're in a lull when cancer isn't on their minds. You can also suggest to older kids that they keep a journal as a way to express their cancer concerns.

RULE #17: WATCH FOR WARNING SIGNS

"Children don't hide their stuff," says Michelle Brauntuch, a child life specialist at Englewood Hospital and Medical Center in New Jersey, who produced a video called *Talking to Your Children About Your Breast Cancer.* If a sound sleeper begins suffering from nightmares or insomnia, if you see your child overeating or not eating at all, if a child grows quiet or acts out—your child is telling you something. And you may need the help of a therapist.

RULE #18: CHECK CANCER PERCEPTIONS REGULARLY

You don't have to give the kids a constant stream of updates, like those tickers that run across the bottom of the CNN screen: Mom's blood count's low; getting shots to bring up blood count; shots really, really hurt. . . . Instead, Brauntuch recalls the example of a dad who would say to his kids every night: "Any questions about Mom? Anything that's confusing or uncertain?" Or sometimes just, "What are you thinking about Mom?" That gives them a chance to express the thoughts and fears that are in their hearts, and lets you tell them what they want to know. Don't be surprised if they ask questions you've already answered, because that's how kids (and a lot of adults) operate.

RULE #19: CHECK IN ABOUT OTHER STUFF, TOO

Ask the kids how their day was and what's going on at school. "In the stress of cancer, ordinary communication could shut down," McCabe cautions. "Kids will resent it if they've had a full day and nobody's asking about it." Even teenagers might wonder why you're not asking about their day, because they've been looking forward to saying, "Dad, shut up!"

RULE #20: KEEP THINGS FUN

Throughout the months of treatment, make sure the kids still have time for fun—play dates, playground visits, movies, whatever distracts them from cancer. You can even turn a moment of trauma into an occasion for laughter. One woman had a pre-chemo head-shaving party with her husband and children, then invited the kids to paint her bald scalp with bright colors.

RULE #21: DON'T PUT YOUR WIFE INTO ISOLATION

"Instead of keeping Mommy behind closed doors," says Dave Como, whose triplets were age 5 at the time, "the kids made her stuff, they took the blanket up to her. Or we brought her down to the couch. We normalized it as much as you can."

Randy Harper's 7-year-old daughter, Casey, went with Mom to chemo one time. Seeing the process up close "took a lot of the fear out of it," says Randy. But if you do have a child who wants to visit the chemo room, don't figure on a full visit. Kids quickly grow bored. Perhaps you can bake cookies with your child to bring to the nurses, then make sure someone can take your child home after a short while.

RULE #22: ASK KIDS FOR HELP—UP TO A POINT

Your children can pitch in, but not if you don't ask. I remember one rainy Saturday afternoon in November, when I was dragging grocery bags into the house after a day of running errands. And the kids were plopped on the couch, watching TV. I was feeling a little sorry for myself (okay, a lot sorry) so I just exploded, "Can't you even help me out?" It seemed to me it was pretty obvious that I needed help, what with my coming in and out of the house and schlepping bags and issuing proclamations such as, "I can't believe how many bags I have to drag in." My 16-year-old listened calmly to my temper tantrum and replied, "Dad, if you ask us, we'll be glad to help."

D'oh.

So I asked, and they helped.

On the other hand, your teenagers shouldn't turn themselves into substitute parental units. "If the dad recognizes that this is happening," says McCue, "address it. Tell your kids, 'I appreciate your help, but I know you have friends, and I want you to find a way to spend time with them.'" And make sure they do.

RULE #23: REMEMBER, KIDS WILL BE KIDS

Your youngsters are not going to be perfect little Buddhas, helpful and good and kind from sunup to sundown. If that's what you think will happen, you're surely in for a big disappointment.

Ken Pruitt used the "Momma first" method to keep his four in line—they were 13, 11, 10, and 7 at the time of Aileen's diagnosis. "As soon as one of them got into a selfish mode, thinking the world revolves around them, I would start chanting, "Momma first" and the others would follow.

And life will be a little easier if you don't wait until things spin out of control. "Try to anticipate," says Frank Sadowski, father of three teenagers and

WHEN THE KIDS AREN'T HOME

A parent's protective instincts never fade. Some moms and dads think that if children are at college or living on their own, there's no need to burden them with news of their mother's breast cancer. But failure to disclose can take a major toll. Odds are that your grown kids will eventually find out what happened. Your wife may then reassure them: "Everything's fine now."

But what will they think the next time they call to see how things are going, and she repeats the same message? It'll be hard for them to believe she's telling the truth.

husband of a breast cancer survivor. "Don't just say to your wife, 'If the kids are bothering you, let me know and I'll go down and shut 'em up.' Plan to take the kids out of the house if you know it's going to be the bad post-chemo afternoon."

RULE #24: DON'T FORGET TO ENJOY YOUR KIDS!

When I visited Steve Romero and Lili Romero-DeSimone at their Alexandria, Virginia, townhouse, they shared some of the trials they'd been through: a mastectomy, chemotherapy, radiation. Then came a magical moment with their 16-month-old daughter Micaela, a real charmer with her saucer eyes, sweet smile, and head full of honey-blond curls. Lili, sprouting a fuzzy new growth of post-chemo hair, and big, burly Steve began to sing a song about hot potatoes and cold spaghetti, with a delightfully silly refrain of "gimme that, gimme that, gimme that food." Micaela joined in. The three of them curled up on the couch as they sang. It was just about the most perfect moment of family harmony and love and happiness—and a reminder that kids can give their parents something that cancer can't touch.

Defusing Family Friction

What to do if parents (hers or yours) are causing tension

Think it's tough telling your kids about the diagnosis? Wait till the time comes to break the news to the folks. Sometimes Mom and Pop don't react quite as you'd hoped.

"My husband's parents never ask me how I'm doing," Linda* told me. "It just blows my mind."

Jillian's* mom almost dropped a dinner dish in the sink when her son-in-law mentioned that Jillian was planning to have reconstruction after her mastectomy. "No, no, no; we'll have none of that," she clucked. "God never intended that."

Wei Chin's* parents didn't even know his wife, Betsy, had breast cancer. She had asked him not to tell. She thought the senior Chins, who lived 1,000 miles away, were too frail to handle the news. Then Betsy's parents sent Wei's mom and dad a Christmas card: "Betsy's chemo is going well," they wrote.

Uh-oh.

Not every family will fall into the various parent traps. If you're fortunate, you, your wife, and both sets of parents will form a strong and loving team in the fight against breast cancer.

As for those who aren't so fortunate, let's put it this way: However the older generation behaves under normal circumstances, that's how they'll probably behave during breast cancer treatment—only multiplied by a factor of 10. And the husband may find himself in an awkward spot. Under normal circumstances, if your wife has a disagreement with her mother or father or another family member, you wisely stay out of it. But what happens when tensions arise during breast cancer treatment? "You have to pick the battles you want to fight, and the timing," advises psychologist Mary Ann McCabe, Ph.D. "Who do you want to take on, and when?"

In the interest of family harmony, the names in this chapter have been changed. But the stories are true.

TELL IT LIKE IT IS

Just as parents may want to shield their children from the news of Mom's cancer, they may have the same instinct to protect their parents. And just as it's a bad idea to conceal from the kids, it's equally foolish to keep secrets from Nana and Pop Pop.

The one exception would be if the parents are truly, truly frail. By which I mean: practically in a coma, suffering from an extraordinarily weak heart, or afflicted by Alzheimer's. Parents with severe emotional problems might also be exempt. But most parents can handle the news. They didn't live into their 60s or 70s or 80s without seeing their share of bad stuff, and they've managed to survive. If there are legitimate concerns about their health, you or your wife, or perhaps one of your siblings, should contact the parent's doctor and ask if he or she can cope with the breast cancer diagnosis.

The alternative—keeping the news in—is almost surely going to backfire. "If you create a dirty little secret," says Patricia Spicer, oncology social worker and coordinator of the breast cancer program for the national organization CancerCare, "it closes your parents out of your life. Someone will slip, and they will find out somehow anyway." She recalls one breast cancer patient who decided not to tell her parents. The woman had to be hospitalized because of an infection during chemo. And who should come to the hospital that very day to visit a sick neighbor? Why, her mother. And who did her mother happen to run into?

You can only imagine how hurt a parent would be in such a

circumstance. Your wife might never hear the end of it: "Why didn't you tell me? I'm your mother. Don't you trust me?"

If your wife wants to conceal, and the two of you have children, ask her, "Wouldn't you want our kids to be open with you?"

Wei Chin no doubt wishes he had asked that question. When his hard-of-hearing father called for an explanation of the Christmas card message, Wei hemmed and hawed, then said he'd call his dad back. He got his wife's blessings to tell all, phoned his parents, and did what he wished he'd done at the start: shared the fact that Betsy had breast cancer.

INATTENTIVE IN-LAWS

What should a husband do if his parents aren't calling his wife? Speak up, or forever hold his peace? Perhaps your parents just aren't that close to their

---

HEAD OFF THE BLAME GAME

When parents cause problems, a husbandly intervention—preferably with wifely permission—can be a force for good. But don't expect any miracles.

Consider the case of Scott* and the blame-casting mother-in-law. His wife's mother wanted to fly from her Florida home to care for her daughter the week following a chemo treatment. Nothing wrong with that. Scott, his wife, Sarah, and their two kids dearly love Gramma Elsa, and Scott was looking forward to a week off from kitchen duty.

There was, however, one catch. In phone conversations, Elsa repeatedly told Sarah that she had too much stress in her life, and that's why she got breast cancer. Which is exactly what a breast cancer patient doesn't want to hear, especially in the middle of chemo. One night when Sarah was away at a cancer support group meeting, Scott called his mother-in-law and told her how glad they were that she was coming but that she couldn't tell Sarah that anything she did, ate, smoked, thought about, or dreamed of had caused her breast cancer. "When you're going through chemo, you need all your strength to get through it," he said, "and you don't want to hear that you've brought it on yourself." Elsa began crying on the phone. So did Scott. When Elsa came to stay, she hewed to the rules.

daughter-in-law and talk to her infrequently. But in a time of crisis, they can certainly pick up the phone every week or so. The obstacle may be fear of not knowing what to say, or of saying the wrong thing. That's no doubt why Zach's* mother would call and sympathize about the plight of "that poor woman"—aka her daughter-in-law—but never seemed to have the time to talk to her.

A son needs to be diplomatic. Social worker Frank McCaffrey—who counsels breast cancer husbands at Boston's Beth Israel Deaconess Medical Center—has seen men raise the subject of avoidance with their parents, only to be rebuffed: "What do you mean? Of course I care!" His suggestion is to try telling your parents that your wife would like to hear from them, then shift the emphasis to yourself: "It's hard for me to know what to say. It must be hard for you, too." Add that all they really need to say is a very low-key, "How are you?"

Maybe the problem is that your parents, or hers, won't *stop* calling. That's

---

But a few weeks after her visit, she was back to her old self. Elsa called her daughter one night and told her she'd just read an article that pinpointed the cause of Sarah's breast cancer. And you'll never guess what it was. Exercise! (Elsa must have been reading the *Bizarro World Journal of Medicine*, because exercise is thought to decrease a woman's risk of developing breast cancer.) Furthermore, Elsa had figured out what type of exercise caused Sarah's cancer—cutting the grass with an old-fashioned reel mower. Clearly, vibrations from the mower had traveled up Sarah's arms and induced a tumor.

So whose fault was it really, when you think about it? Scott's, of course. Because aren't husbands supposed to mow the lawn?

Scott was ready to pick up the phone and tell Elsa how upsetting her new theory was. But then he and Sarah began giggling at the sheer ridiculousness of it. And soon they were guffawing. They laughed until tears ran down their cheeks.

"I didn't make the call," Scott says, still grinning at the memory. "Actually, I should have sent Elsa a thank-you note, because that was the best laugh we'd had in months."

when you can be a gentle buffer, giving an update on how your wife is feeling and adding that she's not up to a phone conversation right that minute.

Or perhaps every time they call they blame your wife for her cancer. Unfortunately, that's how some parents react. Afraid for their child's life, they want to prove that they aren't responsible for causing the disease by, say, failing to make their daughter eat her brussels sprouts. So maybe they'll tell her all the stress in her life caused the cancer.

You or your wife could respond to such an unhelpful remark by simply saying, "You know what? That wasn't helpful," suggests McCabe. Or, she says with a grin, when the unhelpful cancer comments come, just sing a silly song like "Yellow Submarine" in your head.

But a yellow submarine might not go deep enough to evade familial incursions. Poor Diane* was being battered on two fronts. Her mother kept telling her that working too hard caused her cancer. Her sister was a devotee of the deodorant theory—that harmful ingredients in antiperspirants penetrate the armpit and trigger breast cancer (or conversely that antiperspirants prevent body toxins from exiting via sweat). Medical science has found no conclusive evidence to support either the stress or the deodorant thesis, but that didn't matter to Diane's mom and sister. Nor did Diane's protests end their speculations. Her husband asked McCabe for a solution. She proposed: Tell your mother- and sister-in-law that your wife isn't up to hearing such talk, and suggest that instead they talk amongst themselves.

The doom-and-gloom family member is another burden to bear. Barbara* said that every time she talked to her father about her cancer, he made her feel as if she should be picking out a casket. Her solution was to delegate a stand-in. When Barbara's father called, her husband would say she wasn't available. Instead, he'd answer Dad's questions and fill him in on the latest developments. If you're not eager for the job, see if your wife can ask a sibling to stand in.

GUESS WHO'S COMING TO MAKE DINNER?

When a long-distance family member wants to come for an extended visit to "help out in your time of need," you and your wife need to think about the

GUY TALK

"My mom likes to be involved. But my wife just wanted to have me and her own mother in our house during chemo, when she was losing her hair and vomiting. I had to tell my mother, 'This isn't about you and your feelings. It's about what's best for Cindy. If you feel slighted because you are not here, you have to work through that.' "

—AL KNIGHT*, 42
His mom flew in from out-of-town after his wife's diagnosis

ramifications. "Sometimes it works well," McCaffrey tells the breast cancer couple.

And sometimes it doesn't. Your wife may feel as if her parents are treating her like a child again. Your mother or mother-in-law may come in like a bulldozer, re-arranging the kitchen and criticizing the way you run things in your house. "That's not what you're looking for," McCaffrey notes in the understatement of the millennium. "Some parents are very sensitive and can stay out of the way and not disrupt anything. Others take charge in a different way. There's almost always an adjustment."

The last thing your wife needs is to adjust to new arrangements at home. You can calmly point out that your wife is going through a period when she feels that she has lost control over many parts of her life. But her home is one area where she still has control. And what she needs more than anything is for things to be the way they've always been.

If your mother-in-law thinks you're not doing a good job managing things, tell her that you may not be the best household manager in the world, but "it works for us." Better yet, if she's criticizing, say, your laundering skills, try asking, "Would you like to do that? That would be great!"

"Usually, they back off," says social worker Patricia Spicer.

A pre-emptive strike might be useful in some cases, particularly if a blame-casting parent is planning a visit. You can ask your wife's permission to call and lay down some ground rules. Or if you have a good relationship with your in-laws, you might call first and tell your wife later. (But you should tell her, or else her mother might say, "You'll never guess who called me today!")

If a husband does decide to put in a call, he should resist the temptation to rant. "Some husbands say to their in-laws, 'You are wrong and stupid, and you have always been wrong and stupid,'" notes oncology social worker Jill Taylor-Brown. Quash that urge. The point is to talk to them about what would be helpful—and what would most definitely not be helpful—for your wife during a visit.

HER MOTHER, THE DOCTOR

When your wife's parents have opinions about medical treatments, tensions can run even higher. In addition to talking to their daughter, her parents may pull you aside, too. Your job is to assure them that they've been heard—and their daughter will make the decision that she deems best. You can add that, as a breast cancer husband, you don't tell your wife what to do; you respect her right to make treatment decisions. I hope they follow your lead.

But maybe they won't. "I don't think Lee* should have chemo," her mother would say over and over to husband Zach, seeking an ally. Zach would reply (again and again), "I hear what you're saying, but you have to understand that Lee's doctors think chemo will give her the best chance at a long and cancer-free life."

When Jillian's* mom began preaching against reconstruction, Jillian began to wonder—was she doing the right thing? Her mother's comments "threw her for a loop," Ted remembers. "I know your mom means well," he told his wife, "and she's also had breast cancer—but this has got to be your call. I'm going to ask your mom to step back."

And so he did. Jillian had her reconstruction and is quite pleased with the results.

A STERLING SON-IN-LAW

I surely don't mean to imply that the only interactions with your folks and in-laws are going to be fraught with painful moments. Many husbands have sung the praises of a mother-in-law's cooking or been grateful to have help during chemo. Husbands also have told me how touched they were by the love and support shown by both sets of parents.

And your in-laws may be deeply touched by all *you're* doing. "My mom never cared much for Rich," says Tara*. But Rich turned out to be a Grade A breast cancer husband. He came to doctor's appointments and treatments, he was a superb dad to the couple's 16-month-old, and he let Tara know how much he loved her after she lost a breast and her hair. She bragged to her mom about his excellent support, and Mom saw firsthand when she came to visit. "Now," Tara says, "he's my mom's hero."

TIPS ➢ ➢ ➢

1. Tell the parents. How can you and your wife go through a major crisis and hope to conceal it from your folks and her folks?
2. Are your parents afraid to talk to your wife? Tell them you know how hard it is to figure out what to say—but "How are you feeling?" is a good start.
3. Getting unneeded medical advice from your wife's parents? They may think they're saving their daughter's life. Thank them, but tell them that their daughter has faith in her doctors and is confident that she is getting appropriate treatments.

➢ BONUS TIP

If your wife's parents are avoiding her, they need a talking-to. If you've got a good relationship with them, speak up. Or you could ask one of your wife's siblings or a beloved aunt to handle the job. "It doesn't matter who does it, as long as someone does it," advises social worker Jill Taylor-Brown.

Help Wanted: Appointment Pal

Your job at the doctor's office

Every breast cancer patient deserves an appointment pal—someone to accompany her on doctor's visits. There's a good chance that pal will be you.

"If there is a husband in the picture," says Marisa Weiss, M.D., the Philadelphia breast radiation oncologist who is president and founder of breastcancer.org, "it really is useful to come to every initial meeting"—that is, to the first meeting with each of the doctors who will care for your wife. You'll have a face to go with the doctor's name, an impression of his or her manner, and some basic information about what to expect in the weeks and months ahead.

But why stop at first dates? John Davis of Bowie, Maryland, went to doctor's appointments with his wife, Dorothy, whenever he could. Diagnosed with breast cancer 7 years ago, she underwent a mastectomy, followed by reconstructive surgery. "Can you imagine her going, and coming back and telling you what the doctor said?" John asks. "By going with her, you're part of the event. You're not sitting on the sidelines. You learn what she is going to experience."

And just by holding her hand you can make a difference. That gesture is, of course, a tangible sign of love and affection. But it might be a boon in other ways. At the University of North Carolina at Chapel Hill, researchers told 183 couples they'd have to deliver a short speech about something that made them angry. The prospect of public speaking about such an experience was deemed a source of stress. One hundred couples were instructed to hold hands for 10 minutes, then hug for 20 seconds, before the speech. The other 83 couples didn't show the same affection but sat together and waited for their cue. The study findings: The hand-holders' blood pressures and heart rates were significantly lower than those of the couples who didn't hold hands.

So go ahead, be your wife's appointment pal.

That is, unless she tells you not to come.

TO GO OR NOT TO GO

Remember, your wife is the captain of her support team. She's the one who gets to make the final call about who comes along. Maybe you're not the best one to have in a doctor's office.

Norma's* husband was a crier. He tended to shed tears at doctor's visits. Clearly, this was a sign that he loved his wife deeply and was profoundly upset at the thought of losing her. But would anyone want a consistently tearful appointment pal? I don't think so. Neither did Norma. She told him to stay home, and she meant it.

Or perhaps your wife prefers a family member who has special expertise. Lois Hazel, from Bucks County, Pennsylvania, who was diagnosed at age 56, knew the questions she wanted to ask after her breast cancer diagnosis, but she worried that she'd be overcome by emotion. She wanted a good advocate: her sister Carole, a physical therapist. So she told her husband that he didn't have to come to appointments. As Lois puts it, "Dale's not very good with medical issues." And because she talked it over with Dale, he didn't feel as if he'd been cut from the team.

"Lois asked me if I was offended," recalls Dale, 58. "I said, 'No, not at all. I want you to have whatever help is available. If you feel she's the better help, I'm not offended at all.'" Besides, Dale works nights as a truck driver and sleeps during the day; he was grateful that he could keep his schedule intact.

But you do have to ask yourself: Is she telling me to stay away because she feels a little guilty imposing? Frank Sadowski's wife, for example, encouraged him to skip routine consultations and to just drop her off at chemo. He

GUY TALK

"We were always taking our pulse, so to speak, looking back on information we'd gathered, reviewing the information we'd gotten from doctors."

—BRUCE BATHER, 53
Chicago

didn't buy it. A friend and fellow breast cancer husband had told Sadowski, "Whatever she tells you, don't believe it. One thing she wants more than anything else is your physical presence during all this stuff." So Frank went with his wife to every appointment, and that was fine with her.

All you have to do is ask if it's okay if you come anyway. Or just tell her you're coming along, and see how she reacts. Most likely she'll be glad for the company. Otherwise, you might end up like the couple that called the Y-ME breast cancer hotline one night and spoke to breast cancer husband Tom Stern. Here's how he remembers their exchange:

Wife: You're not there when I need you.
Husband: I am.
Wife: You don't come with me to doctor's appointments.
Husband: You don't want me to come.

One thing is certain: If you never come, you risk being shut out of your wife's breast cancer experience. One of the saddest stories I heard about appointment routines comes from nurse care coordinator Anne O'Connor of Georgetown University's Lombardi Cancer Center in Washington, D.C. A breast cancer patient—let's call her Flo—would come for doctor's appointments. Sometimes her husband would bring her; he'd drop her off and pick her up an hour or so later, or sit in the car and wait. On other occasions, her sister brought her. After a time, Flo died of the disease. Following her death, the husband called O'Connor—he'd come across her name in a letter from the hospital—to ask some questions. He wanted to know more about his wife's fight with breast cancer. He said he had encouraged her to seek medical help but that she had shut him out of this part of her life. Still, he didn't seem to be there for her 100 percent—O'Connor remembers when the woman was very ill, her sister brought her to the emergency room, and her husband was nowhere to be seen. So he was far from a perfect husband, and yet he cared enough to call O'Connor after his wife had died.

What could this husband have said, I asked O'Connor, if he had wanted to make amends and if he had wanted to go to the doctor's office with his wife? She offered this advice in hindsight: "My opinion is that he should have said, 'I love you and I need to know what's going on. We're in this together.'"

OFFICE ETIQUETTE

Accompanying your wife to doctor's appointments doesn't automatically earn you a gold star. All of us husbands could stand a lesson in the etiquette of office visits.

We all know about guys and doctors—namely, we don't go as often as we should. Women, on the other hand, typically see their OB-GYNs regularly and take the kids to appointments. They're accustomed to the sometimes glacial pace of a doctor's office. "For some husbands, waiting for visits is a nightmare," says Julia Rowland, Ph.D., the warm and witty psychologist who runs the National Cancer Institute's Office of Cancer Survivorship in Bethesda, Maryland. They're thinking "I've got to get back to work; let's get this over with."

Sitting in the office and fuming when the doctor is running late doesn't help. Deep breathing might. Or a good book. Or *Sports Illustrated*. Or office work. If the delays are endless, ask if you and your wife can go out for coffee and come back in an hour. When our surgeon was delayed at the hospital one time, that's what we did.

Besides, it's not as if the doctor will never show up. Waiting for a doctor is like waiting for a bus. You know the bus is going to come, and you know the doctor is going to see you. Cursing and ranting won't speed things up.

When you and your wife enter the doctor's office, remember: It's not about you. The doctor should give your wife priority in every way. After all, she's the patient. The doc should shake *her* hand first and establish eye contact with her, not you. But that doesn't mean you should lurk in the shadows. Your wife can and should introduce you (or whomever she brings with her) to the doctor, and she might say that she feels comfortable discussing all aspects of her case with you there.

In this era of the HIPAA privacy rule, a breast cancer patient who wants her husband to be able to request information about her case may want to add, "My husband is very involved in my care. I want to make sure he doesn't have any problems getting relevant information. Are there any forms I can sign to facilitate this?" That should cover both regulations from the Health Insurance Portability and Accountability Act of 1996 and any institutional policies, says Susan Bouregy, Ph.D., the chief HIPAA privacy officer at Yale University.

Even if you never utter a word, you're not merely window dressing. On the most elemental level, your very presence in the doctor's office makes a difference. First, let's imagine the scene with no husband or other appointment pal. Just the doctor and the patient. Do I have to tell you who has the power in the room? Hint: It's not your wife. "She's probably wearing no clothes or a shmatte," says Dr. Weiss, who has a clear-eyed view of the man's role at the appointment. Half-naked, clad in an ill-fitting exam-room gown, sitting on an examining table with her feet dangling like a little kid, "she feels diminished and unempowered."

And lonely. I sat in on an appointment at the Johns Hopkins Breast Center in Baltimore when surgeon Ted Tsangaris, M.D., told a divorced woman that she had breast cancer. I was struck by how utterly alone she seemed. Her cancer had been caught early and her treatment was likely to be relatively mild: lumpectomy and radiation, no chemo. The doctor was sympathetic and supportive. But he was still the doctor and she was still the patient—with no one there to hug her, or hold her hand, or cast her a loving glance. As she asked questions, she seemed tentative and nervous.

Just by being there, you change the delicate doctor–patient balance. Instead of almighty doctor > vulnerable patient, the equation is now patient plus pal > doctor: "Having the husband—or another close friend or family member—there can make the woman feel more empowered and confident and ready and willing to ask questions," Dr. Weiss believes. That's an important edge to have. The clock is always ticking at medical appointments, and the patient must be assertive and efficient in her exchanges.

"There are a few doctors who are excellent but sexist," adds Dr. Weiss. "They might be more respectful of the husband because he is a man, and the woman going with a man to such doctors will get more time or more thoughtful, complete answers." That's because men like to show off in front of each other.

The husband can ask questions, too, but be careful how you ask. Some men treat the doctor's visit as an extension of the corporate boardroom. They want to run the appointment as they might run a business meeting. Remember, your wife is the boss. "Ask questions like, 'Can you explain that further?'" Dr. Weiss suggests. "That's different than saying, 'I have a question.' You have to have the woman be in charge, and support her in her role as the patient, rather than take over." A husband who is too bullish or domineering might make the woman feel as if she is stupid. She might end up feeling incapable of asking questions.

Of course, there's an exception to every rule in breast cancer, and the same applies to doctor's appointments. Your wife's coping mechanism may be to allow you to take the lead. Susan Abrams, a Maryland social worker who counsels breast cancer patients, remembers a woman who did not want to hear any information that wasn't absolutely critical for her to hear. At her request, her husband and her sister came to every appointment. They asked the questions; they wrote things down. The woman stayed in the background. At one appointment that would involve no decisions, just information gathering, the patient went to work (which made her feel better) and her husband and sister met with the doctor. The doctor was a little nonplussed. But that's how this patient coped. She was treated with surgery and chemotherapy, and Abrams reports that she's now doing fine.

SOLO ACT

What if you want time alone with the doctor?

Now you're diving into dangerous waters.

"Secrecy and deception only erode what you need most in a crisis—enhanced trust and open communication," says social worker Matthew Loscalzo.

"If you say to the doctor, 'just tell me and don't tell her,' that's setting up a conspiracy," says Dr. Rowland of NCI. "If he's a good doctor, he'd say to the husband, 'I can't talk to you behind her back.'"

But let's say you ask your wife's permission. And she agrees, and informs the doctor that it's okay to talk frankly with her husband. Then the husband is "not acting inappropriately," Dr. Rowland says. Indeed, that's how Larry and Emma Gold* handled the situation when information about Emma's lymph node status seemed distressing. Larry, the eternal pessimist, wanted to ask questions that he feared might unsettle his more upbeat wife. He wanted a clearer sense of her prognosis, and of whether clinical trials or complementary therapies might be beneficial. "She was okay with my asking whatever I wanted to ask," Larry says. "But she agreed it might not be best for her to be there."

"The husband did the right thing by honoring his wife's desire to remain optimistic," Dr. Rowland says. "At the same time, he obtained the information he needed to plan for the future."

Unfortunately, when Larry asked what his wife should do, the doctor gave a flip and cutting response: "Make a will."

So he never told Emma what the doctor said. And that's the risk of any solo visit. You might walk away with knowledge that you feel you must keep to yourself.

GET A JOB DESCRIPTION

To avoid any misunderstandings, you and your wife should have an early discussion about the role she'd like you to play. Ask her: "How can I be most helpful to you when we go to the doctor?"

You can, for example, help her come up with a list of questions before each visit. If that's your job, ask her what she wants to know from this doctor. What statistics does she want to ask about? Have you or she found any information on the Internet that she would like to present for the doctor's point of view? That's how my wife and I functioned. She would tell me the questions she'd want to ask. I'd write them down and bring the list to the appointment. As the visit would draw to a close, I could remind her, "You also wanted to ask about this or that." And you know how much we breast cancer husbands like having our chores to do. If you can't be a Mr. Fix-It, you can at least be the Reminder Guy.

KEEP A RECORD

Then there's the matter of remembering the doctor's answers. And comments. And advice. You'd think that in an hour-long meeting with a doctor discussing a life-threatening disease that afflicts your wife, she would commit every word to memory. In fact, a newly diagnosed breast cancer patient is not a good listener or rememberer. And who can blame her? One day she's feeling fine. The next day, she's living in Cancerland. She may well be in shock.

"We assume that half of what you hear goes in one ear and out the other," says Dr. Rowland. Or maybe even more. In an article called "Patients' memory for medical information," published in the *Journal of the Royal Society of Medicine* in May 2003, neuropsychology professor Roy Kessels, Ph.D., from Utrecht University in the Netherlands reported on relevant studies: "Forty-to-eighty percent of medical information provided by health care practitioners is forgotten immediately." The more information presented, the less a patient remembers. And what the patients do recall is often incorrect. The aging process makes it worse. So does anxiety. After a doctor says, "You have *x* disease, and this will affect everyday activities for the rest of your life," writes Dr. Kessels, that may be when the patient stops listening.

An obvious solution to the problem of patient shutdown is to tape-record key appointments. That way, you and your wife have a record of what the doctor said. The polite way of handling this is to ask permission. (One presumptuous patient already had the recorder running when Dr. Marisa Weiss entered the room.) But if you ask, you should get a "yes." A doctor who is not comfortable being recorded may not be the kind of doctor you wish to see.

It's practically a scientific fact that men like technology more than women do, so you may end up being the keeper of the recorder. I suggest packing a spare tape and backup batteries in your jacket pocket.

But the 21st century woman can operate a recorder on her own, and she may have more room for all the apparatus in her purse. Besides, if you're unable to make a key appointment, she can use the recorder to keep you in the loop. Olympia Cotto had to see her oncologist on a day when her husband could not get off from work. She taped the doctor's explanation of the impact of chemotherapy on her fertility. And the impact wasn't good—a 70 percent chance of ovarian dysfunction. "I was very depressed," she recalls of the visit 6 years ago. "We were trying to have a baby. I thought, 'This is going to put an end to our marriage.'"

When she got home, she gave her husband the tape—and left the room. She couldn't bear to watch. "What do you think?" she later asked. He said, "I don't care about ovarian dysfunction—I want to have you around."

If you and your wife don't relish the thought of listening to tapes of a doctor's comments, there's always pen and notepad. There it is, in black and white—assuming you can read your scrawlings. Don't be embarrassed to ask the doctor to repeat a statement to make sure that you've jotted it down correctly.

By serving as the note taker, a husband can give his wife the freedom to look the doctor in the eye and watch the doctor's body language. Then again, I have also spoken to women with breast cancer who were reporters, and they diligently took notes just as they had for years in their job. Just make sure that you figure out together who will do what at the doctor's office. One of you can also ask the physician for what Dr. Kessels calls in his study a "visual communication aid." My wife's surgeon drew a rudimentary sketch of a breast on a sheet of paper, pinpointed the tumor, then jotted down a few relevant facts about its makeup. Nothing beats an old-fashioned, take-home cheat sheet—far more effective than video or multimedia presentations, Dr. Kessels concludes.

READ HER REACTION

In case you haven't noticed, your potential job responsibilities are growing by the minute: giver of moral support, note taker, keeper of the question list. In addition, you should pay close attention to your wife's reaction to the information. Think of yourself as an emotional radar monitor. You're the only one who might catch the wave of fear or panic that sweeps across your wife's face, and you're the only one who can reassure her. "Greg would have a different spin coming out of appointments," remembers his wife Heidi LaFleche. "He was more rational; he saw the whole picture. The doctor may have said five positive things and one negative thing. I would remember the one negative. The doctor might have said, 'Only 1 percent of people who take Adriamycin have heart failure.'" To Heidi that meant: "I'll stick my arm out for chemo and die." And Greg would bring her back to reality.

WORKPLACE WORRIES

If you do plan to be your wife's appointment pal, you'll need to give a heads-up to the folks at the office. In the first few weeks after diagnosis, you're going to be missing half days and whole days—and you may have to vanish at a moment's notice, because that's just how breast cancer is. And then comes chemotherapy.

I hope your boss tells you to take as much time as you need. That's what you want to hear, because there's a lot of time involved. Getting to the appointment, waiting around because the doc is running late, listening intently during the period that you have the doctor's undivided attention, then going over the information with your wife. True, it can be hard to disappear from work for hours at a time on a regular basis. But it's not impossible. "The company was unbelievable," says Frank Sadowski, vice president for consumer electronics merchandising at amazon.com. "I just did it," remembers Stephen Peck. "My boss was understanding. But if he wasn't, I still would have taken off."

That's easy for him to say. Some employers really do make it damned difficult for the husband. Richard Robert, who is a federal law enforcement agent, had over 700 hours of sick leave—more than enough to take his wife, Suzanne, to all her appointments. And Richie didn't want to miss one. "I just didn't want her to be by herself, getting bad news. I wanted to be there to listen, to be able to help her make decisions, to gather information, to see and to hear, like a copilot." On long drives to and from the doctor's office, he wanted to be with her because "she needs somebody to share the good times and bad times. I wouldn't want her to get really emotional and down-and-out by herself." He also didn't want her to quietly accept all that the doctor said. "It's just not her nature to ask a doctor questions," he adds. "But she didn't mind if I did." He thinks that her reticence stems from her heritage. She's from Guam, he explains, where people "tend to idolize the doctors almost like demigods. So they never ask questions: It's rude, you're questioning his integrity." (As a footnote, I'd add that plenty of non-Guamanians have the same approach.)

At any rate, Richie went with his wife to every appointment, every chemotherapy session, every blood test or x-ray. His boss began asking for documentation. "He probably was thinking this guy has got to be screwing off," Richie says. His wife's doctor wrote a letter of support saying that "a spouse or loved one's involvement is key to recovery. He has been here every time. I support his being here with his wife." Nonetheless, memos went into his file, and at one point his pay was docked. Eventually, Richie filed a discrimination complaint—he was the only Puerto Rican agent in the division and felt that anti-Latino sentiment played into the situation. "There was a settlement," he says. "I'm not supposed to talk about it. But I felt vindicated by the terms of the settlement."

Richie has a lot of guts. I asked the folks at the Patients Advocate Foundation about the options for a husband who gets the message that he shouldn't be taking time off for his wife's medical matters. The Family and Medical Leave Act should guarantee you the right to accompany a spouse on appointments about cancer; but the spokeswoman I talked to admitted that once you file a complaint, you risk poisoning the atmosphere at work beyond repair.

That's why some breast cancer husbands decide to keep their wife's disease a secret, using sick days or personal days so they can attend important appointments and treatments, and calling on family and friends to lend a hand. "I used to recommend that everybody be honest, at least with their immediate supervisors," says Hester Hill Schnipper, chief of oncology social work at Boston's Beth Israel Deaconess Medical Center. "I think that's mostly true, but I understand there are some workplaces where that is a mistake because of job security. Yes, there are laws about discrimination, but you can never prove that's the reason if there are repercussions for missing time."

Schnipper does offer a cautionary note: "Think about why you're not disclosing. Is it because you're embarrassed or because they'll screw you at work if they know?"

Then there are the men who do tell their bosses, only to have it made clear that too much time off is not acceptable.

Mike Malone was working for an ad agency in San Francisco when his bride-to-be was diagnosed with breast cancer. He wanted to go with her for her chemo treatments. "You just hope for the reaction most people get—take the day." Instead, his boss's response was more like, "Take the hour." So Mike would leave Stacy's chemo treatments early to head back to work. "But there

---

A SUPREMELY KIND HUSBAND

Even a Supreme Court justice needs an appointment pal. When Sandra Day O'Connor was diagnosed in 1988, she was stunned by the impact of the news. "I was unprepared for the enormous emotional jolt from that diagnosis," she says. And she couldn't believe she had to make treatment decisions so quickly. She had oral arguments she needed to hear; she thought she might have a couple of months to mull things over. "I was told this was not an option. I lacked an appreciation that everything had to stop and I had to focus on my health problem."

Only she found she couldn't focus. "I decided I needed ears other than my own," she says. "I was so emotionally involved. I wasn't sure I was hearing everything."

O'Connor asked her husband to come with her to her doctor's appointments—so he could take notes and listen carefully to what the doctors had to say. "The diagnosis is devastating," she says, "and I think the person with cancer doesn't hear things totally or objectively. His help that way was terribly important."

John O'Connor was more than happy to oblige. "He was," she says, "very, very helpful."

He continued to be her support as she went through chemotherapy, taking her to the appointments and driving her home afterward when she was feeling shaky. "During the course of treatment, it's so important to have support from somebody who cares," she says. "It makes an enormous difference in your capacity to deal with cancer."

was a silver lining," he says. Family and friends had offered to do whatever they could to assist. "It's not often that you can say, 'Okay, I can use your help.' It made them feel good."

Mike ended up switching jobs after the ordeal. So did Wei Chin*. "I was in a terrible employment situation," says Chin, a scientist who worked in a research lab at the time. "My boss was furious that I wanted to attend my wife's surgery. It was just awful," recalls Chin, who eventually changed jobs. "I had to move beyond it, or otherwise you just destroy yourself ruminating that there could be such bad people."

NO REGRETS

That should be the motto of the appointment pal, as I see it. Trust me—you're not going to look back and say, "I sure didn't need to go to that doctor's appointment." But you might well be sorry if you don't show up. Because even a routine visit can take unexpected twists, and your wife might be very glad you came along.

That lesson was reinforced one cold, crisp February night. My wife, nearing the end of her 5 months of chemo, had begun experiencing shortness of breath. Her primary care doc was worried enough to order a CAT scan. This was late on a Friday afternoon. Marsha would have to go to a nearby hospital, check in at the emergency room, and wait for the test to be done. "Stay home," Marsha told me. "I'll be fine." I was tempted. It had been a long week—both on the work front and the cancer front—and I was tired. The hospital was just 10 minutes away, so it wasn't a big deal for Marsha to get there on her own. And a scan is just a scan. But something made me say, "I'll come."

We left the house around 7:30 P.M. Marsha waited an interminably long time just to be seen by a doctor . . . And then to have a technician perform the scan . . . And to get feedback from a radiologist. It was 9:00 P.M. . . . 10:00 P.M. . . . 11:00 P.M. We were bored out of our skulls. We made jokes about the doctors and nurses. We read old issues of *Good Housekeeping*. As we waited, we'd set deadlines: If no one comes to us in the next 15 minutes, we're checking with the head nurse. Okay, we're giving them 10 more minutes before we nag. None of our reminders made a difference. In fact, the whole evening didn't seem to make much of a difference in terms of figuring out what was wrong with Marsha. The CAT scan didn't show any obvious problems that might be causing the shortness of breath. By the time we got home, it was way past midnight, and we were both suffering from shortness of sleep and patience.

But I wasn't sorry I went. Marsha was grateful to have my company, and I would have felt like a heel if she had spent those 5 hours alone. And it wasn't a total loss. After all, how often does a married couple with kids get 5 whole hours alone together? As we staggered wearily up the front sidewalk in the wee hours of Saturday morning, I turned to Marsha, grabbed her hand, and said, "See honey, you can't say we never go out anymore!"

TIPS ➢ ➢ ➢

1. Go with a list of questions. Star the ones that are most urgent. And find out if the doctor will reply to queries via e-mail if time runs out in the office.
2. Don't leave the doctor's office without a clear sense of what's been said. At the end of the appointment, you or your wife should ask the doctor to review recommendations—the why and the wherefore.
3. Is your wife visiting the doc for the first time? Volunteer to call ahead and ask what she should bring—mammogram films, medical records. Then pack them up and bring them along. It's one less thing for her to worry about.

➢ BONUS TIP

Is a doctor not taking time to answer your wife's questions? Maybe it's time to find another doctor. When Linda Ellerbee's surgeon tired of her queries, he said—as Ellerbee remembers it—"You know, there's this doctor Susan Love. Why don't you read her breast cancer book and then you won't have to annoy me with your questions."

"I have a better idea," Ellerbee replied. "Why don't I call this Susan Love, and she can be my surgeon." And that's exactly what she did.

Part II

Treatment and Beyond

Surgical Options

A crash course for husbands

As you no doubt know by now, there are two surgical treatments for breast cancer: lumpectomy (followed by radiation) or mastectomy. Sounds pretty simple. I figured my wife would go to a surgeon, the surgeon would look at all the relevant data and make a recommendation, and that would be that.

Boy, was I ever wrong.

My wife heard a variety of opinions from a variety of surgeons, which is actually a fairly common turn of events for breast cancer patients. And there isn't always a clear-cut "best" choice.

As if that's not confusing enough, I was unsure about my role as the breast cancer husband. I felt as if my job should be to choose the top doctor and a surefire treatment plan for Marsha. Because, after all, aren't husbands supposed to look out for their wives?

I soon came to understand that wasn't my job at all. Marsha had to select a surgeon who made her feel confident, and a surgical option that made sense to both the doctor and to her. But that doesn't mean I sat idly by. I came to realize that I did have a function. I could serve as my wife's sounding board. And that's not just busy work. When a woman asks her husband for affirmation about a doctor or a treatment plan, and he can give it, that's very useful. "If a patient has an echo, a foil, it makes it much easier, even if she may not take the spouse's advice," says oncologist Fred Smith, M.D., who practices in Chevy Chase, Maryland. That's a rule that holds true throughout the cancer experience. Nor should you feel bad if your wife doesn't follow your suggestions. Think of your workplace. You may propose ideas to your boss all the time. The boss will listen, and maybe even thank you. But in the end, the boss will do what the boss wants to do.

Of course, you do know what you're talking about at work. And you probably aren't quite as expert in the breast cancer arena. To be your wife's support guy, you can be more helpful if you know a little about the disease—and about the fine art of selecting a surgeon.

A SURGICAL PRIMER

At the time of diagnosis, neither you nor your wife is likely to speak the language of the disease. "As you know, it's a new world," says Ed Reynolds, 66, of Spokane, Washington, whose wife, Jan, was diagnosed 3 years ago. "You're entering into the unknown." And just about everything that happens is a surprise.

I remember those bewildering days of trekking from surgeon to surgeon and being hit over the head with terms that seemed to have arrived from another planet: sentinel node biopsy, ductal carcinoma, lobular . . . I felt as if I'd stumbled into a college lecture hall I'd never seen before on the day of an exam.

Some excellent books can remedy your ignorance, starting with *Dr. Susan Love's Breast Book*. Her Web site, www.susanlovemd.com, and another site, www.breastcancer.org, are also superb resources. The latter site has a talking dictionary that speaks and defines the terms your wife (and you) will run across in your cancer-a-thon. (You may also find helpful the glossary on page 295.)

Here are a few of the things I wish I had known before I walked into the doctor's office.

The tumor. Aka the lesion or the lump. Tumors have a variety of traits. The most obvious is size, which will be stated in centimeters. For example, a tumor might be 2.1 centimeters, which is the size of . . . okay, at the time,

I didn't know the answer. The best guide I've seen is the Susan G. Komen Breast Cancer Foundation handout that compares tumors to coins—2.1 centimeters is roughly equivalent to a quarter, for example.

Smaller is usually better, for the obvious reasons. But not always. "You can have a small cancer that behaves like a bully, or a large cancer that is

---

SIZING UP A TUMOR

A breast tumor is measured in centimeters: for example, 1.3 or 2.7 or 3.9. For those of us who aren't metric-minded, the Susan G. Komen Breast Cancer Foundation has coined this helpful visual aid.

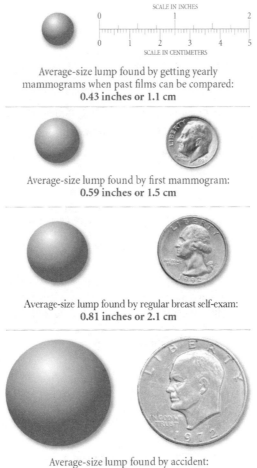

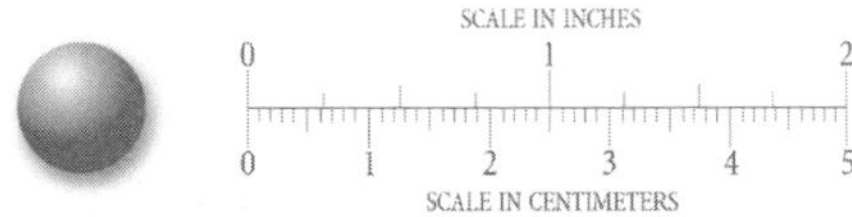

Average-size lump found by getting yearly mammograms when past films can be compared:
0.43 inches or 1.1 cm

Average-size lump found by first mammogram:
0.59 inches or 1.5 cm

Average-size lump found by regular breast self-exam:
0.81 inches or 2.1 cm

Average-size lump found by accident:
1.40 inches or 3.6 cm

mild-mannered," says Marisa Weiss, M.D., the Philadelphia breast radiation oncologist who founded breastcancer.org.

Mild-mannered cancer would be "in situ." The bullying kind is labeled "invasive" or "infiltrating." A tumor could consist of in situ cancer cells, invasive cells, or a mix of the two.

"In situ" is a Latin phrase that simply means "in the site of." The cancer is confined to the ducts or lobules where it began. (The ducts are milk passages, the lobules are milk-producing glands; cancer present in both places is called "mammary.") As long as the cancer is in situ, it has not gone anywhere else in the body. Thus, chemotherapy, which wipes out cancer cells that have traveled from the breast to other parts of the body, is not needed

---

ON STAGES

Your wife will be assigned a "stage"—a category that describes how advanced her cancer is. The stage is based upon the characteristics of the cancer, the size of the tumor, and whether the cancer has spread to lymph nodes or beyond. Your wife's breast cancer stage helps her oncologist determine her course of treatment as well as her prognosis—the most likely outcome of the disease.

STAGE 0

Non-invasive breast cancer (aka carcinoma) in situ. Abnormal or precancerous cells are in the lining of a lobule or a duct, but there is no evidence of cancer cells breaking through to or invading neighboring normal tissue within the breast.

STAGE I

Stages I through IV are all considered invasive breast cancer, which means that cancer cells are breaking through to or invading neighboring normal tissue within the breast.

In stage I, the tumor is fairly small in size, measuring up to 2 centimeters. No lymph nodes are involved.

STAGE IIA

The tumor measures between 2 and 5 centimeters but has not spread to the lymph nodes under the arm on the side of the tumor, or the tumor is smaller than 2 centimeters but has spread to the nodes, or there is no tumor found in the breast but there is cancer in the nodes.

STAGE IIB

The tumor is between 2 and 5 centimeters and has spread to the nodes, or is larger than 5 centimeters but has not spread to the nodes.

for a patient with in situ cancer. But that doesn't mean such a patient can sit back and do nothing. "In 70 percent of women with DCIS [ductal carcinoma in situ], it will turn into invasive cancer," is how breast surgeon Cynthia Drogula, M.D., of Washington, D.C., put it in a conversation with a patient. "There's research going on to see which DCIS will grow into invasive cancers. But it's not going to be available for 7or 8 years—too late for you. We have to assume we're dealing with invasive cancer, and that it has to be removed."

Invasive breast cancer has broken out of its ductal or lobular birthplace. Over time, it can grow in size within the breast; cancer cells can also migrate to other parts of the body. Four out of five breast cancers diagnosed today are

---

STAGE IIIA

The tumor measures larger than 5 centimeters, or cancer cells have spread to lymph nodes under the arm, and nodes are clumping or sticking to one another or surrounding tissue.

STAGE IIIB

Regardless of tumor size, cancer has spread to the breast skin, chest wall, or internal mammary lymph nodes (located beneath the breast inside the chest). This stage includes inflammatory breast cancer, a rare but serious and aggressive cancer whose distinguishing feature is redness on part or all of the breast.

STAGE IIIC

Regardless of tumor size, cancer has spread to lymph nodes under the arm and breastbone, or under and above the collarbone.

STAGE IV

Regardless of tumor size, cancer has spread beyond the breast, underarm, and internal mammary lymph nodes to other sites in the body such as the lungs, liver, bones, or brain. Stage IV is referred to as distant or metastatic disease.

Source: Adapted with permission from www.breastcancer.org, a nonprofit organization that provides in-depth information about breast cancer.

GUY TALK

"My wife had multiple surgeries, for removal of her breast, reconstruction, and then for the recall of her silicone implant. It was enough to send anybody into a tailspin. And she was beaten down by radiation, which really tired her. But she was just stoic about it. There's a myth that men are the strong gender and women are the weak. Well, I think it's the other way around."

—JACK BURLINGAME, 49
Hingham, Massachusetts

invasive. But don't panic: Doctors have devised many treatments to increase patients' chances of living a long and healthy life.

The gravest type of invasive cancer is inflammatory breast cancer. Its rapid spread makes it the most dangerous of breast cancers. This uncommon variation affects only 1 out of every 100 women diagnosed with invasive breast cancer. The signs are striking: red and warm skin on the breast, skin that resembles the peel of an orange. Mammograms have a hard time picking up inflammatory breast cancer because it starts in the skin and grows inward; the condition is often misdiagnosed as mastitis—a breast inflammation sometimes found among nursing mothers.

For just about every newly diagnosed patient, surgery is necessary to remove the cancer. And your wife must make a decision about what kind of surgery to undergo.

One exception: If a tumor has grown very large and the cancer has spread throughout the body, it may be too late to consider surgery as a first-line treatment. "If there is metastatic disease, then one must consider carefully whether to do any surgery," explains William Goodson, M.D., senior clinical research scientist at the California Pacific Medical Center Research Institute and one of the first surgeons in the United States to specialize in breast care. "Out-of-control breast cancer on the chest wall is an awful and ugly thing. If there is a lot of tumor, one may choose to debulk it before doing some sort of radiation therapy. It is a very individual thing."

Lumpectomy is the removal of the lump and a margin of healthy tissue around the lump to ensure that no cancer remains. It is also known as breast conservation, because your wife gets to keep her breast. As you might guess, a woman with a small tumor—say, 4 centimeters or less—is often a good candidate for lumpectomy.

But—you knew there would be a "but" or two—if the tumor is small and your wife's breasts are very small, the surgeon may not be able to perform a lumpectomy. Conversely, if your wife is large-breasted, the surgeon may be able to perform a lumpectomy even if the tumor is relatively large. Some women with larger tumors undergo chemotherapy first to shrink the tumor. If the chemo drugs work, then the patient may be able to undergo a lumpectomy instead of a mastectomy.

The location of the tumor might mean a lumpectomy is not advisable. If the lesion is very close to the chest wall or the nipple, for example, a lumpectomy could be difficult or even impossible to perform. If your wife has several small tumors ("multifocal disease," as it is called), she would not be a good candidate for breast conservation. Even a set of suspicious calcifications or precancerous cells may call for mastectomy, since there is no "lump" to remove; rather, there are potential cancers in a number of spots.

A lumpectomy takes an hour or two to perform. The surgeon draws a line on your wife's breast with a marker indicating the location of the tumor, then slices along the line and peels the skin back to reveal breast tissue. The surgery is something like an excavation—like pulling back the upper layer of turf on your lawn and probing for the roots of a weed in the soil below. The surgeon cuts out the lesion, puts it in a plastic bag and sends it to the pathologist to examine. The surgeon also removes samples of tissue surrounding the tumor—the margins. If the margins are clear—that is, if they test negative for cancer—then the lumpectomy is considered a success and no further surgery will be required.

You'll find out the status of the margins a couple of days after the surgery. If the margins are positive, that doesn't mean mastectomy is automatically the next step. There's nothing wrong with trying a second time for clear margins, as long as the surgeon thinks it's worth a shot. "Good surgeons go back for margins all the time," says Dr. Drogula. "I went back three times for margins with one patient. She was interested in keeping her breast, and we just had one margin we were chasing." Surgeons may disagree on just how much tissue needs to be removed and deemed "clear" of cancer. Depending on the doctor's views and the characteristics of your wife's cancer, the range can be from 1 millimeter to 1 centimeter of surrounding tissue. But there is agreement about one thing: Positive margins are not acceptable.

When the lumpectomy is complete, the surgeon neatly sews up the incision and covers it with Steri-Strips. Soon after the surgery is over, your wife will begin awakening from her anesthesia-imposed slumber.

Radiation. Lumpectomy alone is not a satisfactory treatment choice. With a lumpectomy, your wife will face a 40 percent chance of a local recurrence—that is, of another tumor developing in the same breast. The solution to this dilemma is to marry lumpectomy with radiation, which cuts the odds of recurrence by two-thirds. A radiation oncologist will devise a plan to bombard the breast with x-rays every weekday for a period of 5 to 7 weeks. Radiation destroys any microscopic cancer cells that may remain in the breast after surgery, lowering the chance of local recurrence to around 10 percent. In other words, out of 100 women who undergo this dual treatment, 10 of them will face a local recurrence—a little higher than the typical risk of local recurrence for early-stage patients who have a mastectomy (unbelievable as it may seem, cancer can recur on the chest wall or scar even if no breast remains). Yet even with their slightly higher risk of local recurrence, women who undergo lumpectomy plus radiation have a long-term prognosis, or survival rate, that's the same as women who have a mastectomy.

Because lumpectomy must be paired with radiation, certain patients aren't considered for the breast-conserving surgery. Anyone who previously has had radiation treatment to the breast isn't a candidate for a second round of radiation. That's too much x-ray treatment. In addition, a patient who has a connective tissue disease, like scleroderma, may have no choice but mastectomy. For such women, radiation treatment could trigger distressing side effects.

Mastectomy, or complete removal of the affected breast, is the other surgical option for treating breast cancer. Not too long ago, it was the only option. Although the surgery is more traumatic than lumpectomy for many women, it is in fact a bit more straightforward in the operating room. No need to worry about clear margins. Drains are inserted to handle bodily fluids that build up. The woman is kept in the hospital overnight, or sometimes sent home the same day. (See the chapter titled Missing a Breast on page 140 for more information on mastectomy and its aftermath.)

NODE NEWS

If your wife has invasive breast cancer, the breast surgeon often will take a sample of lymph nodes from her armpit to see if the cancer has spread—that procedure is known as an axillary dissection. For most patients, armpit lymph nodes are the first place breast cancer is likely to spread. The status of the nodes plays a part in the treatment plan. If even one node tests positive for cancer, chemotherapy is recommended.

In the axillary dissection, the doctor makes a cut in the armpit, peels back the skin, and removes a batch of nodes—a sampling might be as small as six or as large as 50. The range is usually 10 to 20. The mastectomy patient's nodes are usually accessed via the same incision made for the mastectomy. The pathologist checks the nodes for cancer and files his report a couple of days after the surgery.

Following a full axillary dissection, your wife will have a bulb-shaped drain dangling from her armpit to collect lymphatic fluid that would otherwise have drained through the now-missing nodes. She may experience numbness in her armpit. And the surgery puts her at lifelong risk for lymphedema—a swelling of the arm and/or hand that can occur if lymphatic fluid doesn't drain properly when there is an infection or other stressor. In the final chapter of this book, The New Normal on page 272, you will find out how you can help your wife stave off lymphedema.

Sentinel node biopsy is a newer procedure that could help your wife avoid an extensive axillary dissection and its unpleasant side effects. If breast cancer cells have moved through lymphatic vessels from the breast to the armpit, the first nodes they would reach are the "sentinel nodes." The average patient has two such nodes; they're often next to each other. If the sentinel node or nodes are cancer-free, the assumption is that the surgeon need not remove additional nodes.

A doctor finds the sentinel nodes by injecting a blue dye or a radioactive material into the breast, either at the tumor site or near the nipple. If all goes well, the dye or the radioactivity will wend its way through the same lymphatic vessels that cancer cells would use in their travels. The sentinel node or nodes can then be identified by color or by a gamma probe. The surgeon removes the sentinel node or nodes early in the surgery.

In a surgery I watched at Johns Hopkins Breast Center in Baltimore, I felt as if I were watching a paint-by-numbers operation. Surrounded by red blood and yellow fat, the blue-stained lymphatic vessel slid around a muscle, and led to the first sentinel node, which looked like a blue jelly bean. The surgeon removed the node, and a nurse dropped it in a plastic bag. Off it went to the pathologist, who froze it and did a quick read. Fifteen minutes or so into the surgery, the preliminary word came back: negative for cancer. No more armpit excavation for this patient. If this initial test reveals a positive node, the surgeon will take a larger sampling of nodes to see how much the cancer has spread.

The sentinel node procedure doesn't always work. "In a certain group of women, we're not going to find the sentinel node," says Ted Tsangaris, M.D., chief of breast surgery at the Hopkins breast center. He estimates the failure rate at less than 5 percent. Among the reasons: unexpected drainage routes or an injection that just didn't work. In addition, if the woman has scattered small tumors in her breast, a sentinel node dissection might not be advisable; the cancer cells could be migrating via different channels.

Furthermore, not every surgeon has the experience to do a sentinel node dissection. Typically, a doctor needs to have done about 30 to 50 surgeries removing the sentinel node and also performing an axillary dissection as a check, to make sure that the finding for the sentinel node matches the findings for the other nodes. The first surgeon my wife saw at our HMO told her that he does the sentinel node procedure (whew, what a relief). But then he added that he automatically does an axillary dissection as well as a backup. I'm all for helping doctors achieve competency in the sentinel node area, but my wife wanted a surgeon who had had enough sentinel node experience to be reasonably confident of success. A breast surgeon is far more likely to have reached that level of expertise than a general surgeon. And the doctor should be able to tell you, "In the past year, I've done 31 sentinel node procedures, and I've found the node in 30 cases." Or some similarly reassuring statistic.

After sentinel node surgery, your wife may be a little blue—literally. If the surgeon uses blue dye to mark the sentinel node, her skin may take on a bluish caste, as will her urine and stool. The color will fade in a day or so. But it did prompt one good-natured patient to burst out in song, "Am I blue?" while her husband broke out in an embarrassed grin.

There is one more thing to mention about sentinel node procedures: in 1 out of 10 cases, the first report on the sentinel node is not correct. The pathologist routinely does another, more thorough study and may find cancer where there seemed to be none. That's the kind of phone call no one wants to get. But it is part of the up-and-down breast cancer experience, where things change for the worse (and sometimes for the better). Whether you're an optimist or pessimist at heart, all you can do is cope with the news and move ahead. In the wake of a false reading for the sentinel node, the doctor may want to perform a full dissection to find out how many nodes are involved. Or not—it depends on how much of the cancer is in the sentinel node. In any case, the nodes will be radiated to treat the cancer.

For certain women, doctors may say that axillary dissection is not necessary. If the tumor is "locally advanced" (aka large), some doctors may think the node sampling doesn't tell a lot, since the size of the tumor alone would already mean that chemotherapy is indicated. In fact, chemo is typically recommended for patients with a tumor 1 centimeter or larger, even if the nodes are negative. If your wife's nodes are palpable—swollen from cancer cells—then the doctor might believe that it is pointless to perform a sentinel node procedure, because the cancer is surely in the armpit. Others disagree. Determining the extent of the spread in the armpit nodes may argue for more aggressive radiation of that area, they say.

At the other end of the scale, some doctors say the nodes needn't be checked if the tumor is very small—say, under 5 millimeters. But even then, the doctor or your wife may want to find out how her nodes look just to know for certain that all is (or isn't) well.

CHOOSING A SURGEON

Now you know a bit about what your wife's surgeon will be doing. But how do you know that your wife has found a surgeon with the appropriate skills to treat her cancer?

"You don't want to go to a surgeon who does an occasional breast operation," says surgeon Katherine Alley, M.D., medical director of the Suburban Breast Center in Bethesda, Maryland, "because a lot of surgery is experience." A surgeon whose practice consists, to a large degree, of breast cancer patients will be in a better position to recommend and perform the appropriate surgery, and to do it deftly. How does one get to be a breast specialist? The doctor may have completed a fellowship specializing in breasts or early in his or her career, may have joined a practice that handles a large number of breast surgeries.

A breast specialist's expertise and experience can benefit your wife in several ways. The specialist may be able to make a smaller incision for a lumpectomy and may be confident that a lumpectomy instead of a mastectomy will be an appropriate surgical treatment. A surgeon less skilled in breast surgery may be more likely to recommend mastectomy. In fact, according to surveys, some breast cancer patients in the United States aren't even told about the option of lumpectomy plus radiation.

Conversely, a breast surgeon might recognize when a mastectomy is needed instead of a lumpectomy. Case in point: A general surgeon performed a bilateral lumpectomy on 34-year-old Suzanne Robert 6 years ago, saying that mastectomy wasn't necessary because "I think we got everything." An oncologist's concerns about the pathology report led to a referral to the Comprehensive Cancer Center at City of Hope in Duarte, California. Suzanne and husband Richard drove 54 miles from their Irvine, California, home to see the director of oncologic surgery, who told them, as Richie remembers, "I believe that your surgeon made a number of errors. Based on the size of the tumors and aggressiveness of the cancer, a bilateral mastectomy should have been done." A month after her bilateral lumpectomy, Suzanne had a bilateral mastectomy.

There's no magic trick to finding out how many breast cancer patients a doctor treats. Just ask. "Nobody should be embarrassed to ask about a doctor's résumé and credentials," says Dr. Drogula. "Ask point blank, what percent of your practice is breast? How many do you do a month, a year, and how long have you been in practice? I wouldn't want someone whose practice was only 10 percent breast. But 50 percent breast, that's a lot of time to devote to breast cancer, if you think about it."

If the answer doesn't sit right with your wife, she should seek another surgeon. Your community may have a hospital with a breast center; she can call and ask for recommendations, or you can volunteer to do the research. The National Cancer Institute in Bethesda, Maryland, can also provide a list of designated cancer centers (800–422–6237 or www.cancer.gov). Because breast cancer is not a rare disease, friends and neighbors will undoubtedly share their recommendations—which is how my wife found her truly wonderful surgeon.

If you can't find a breast specialist in your community, you may want to take a road trip to the nearest big city that has a breast specialist. At the Johns Hopkins Breast Center in Baltimore, I met a patient who had driven an hour from the town of Westminster, Maryland, for her surgery. Of course, your wife will need to visit her surgeon for follow-ups after surgery, and for checkups. But she (and you) may feel that it is well worth the extra time and expense.

Your wife's insurer may not want to pay for the breast surgeon she wishes to see. That's what happened to my wife, because we were HMO members at the time, and the roster of doctors did not include a breast specialist. A competent general surgeon can certainly perform a lumpectomy or mastectomy. But you might consider paying out of pocket to visit a breast specialist just to make sure the general surgeon's recommendation about surgery is appropriate.

If there is a discrepancy in opinions, or if your wife wants to be treated by an out-of-network doctor, then start gathering information. Perhaps there is something about the nature of your wife's disease that argues for a breast specialist—the location of the tumor, for example.

Speaking to a case manager at the insurance company could produce a better result than haranguing the clerk who answers the phone. Your chances of success are not as low as you might think. A study by the Rand Corporation, the nonprofit think tank, looked at cases where a patient appealed for additional services: 42 percent of the time, the patient won. My wife and I, however, were on the verge of losing, with repeated rejections of our request to go out of network for the surgery. Then a health-care-savvy friend suggested that Marsha tell her story to her employer's benefits honcho—how the HMO surgeon had missed a second tumor, how the HMO docs consistently recommended mastectomy while a breast specialist in private practice was an advocate of lumpectomy, if that was Marsha's wish. "I've heard enough," the benefits head said. A sympathetic bureaucrat, she transferred my wife to a more flexible insurance option "for cause," noting that she'd listened to too many stories about substandard care for cancer patients at the HMO.

LISTENING TO THE DOCTOR

Credentials and experience are obviously very important to consider when choosing a surgeon. But so is the surgeon's bedside manner. As you make the rounds of surgeons, you and your wife need to think carefully about what each one says and how he or she relates to your wife. Since she is no doubt in a little more shock than you are, you may be the better listener. But what are you listening for?

A surgeon should be able to explain breast cancer in a way that you can understand. He or she should tell you why a certain surgery is recommended. The doctor's manner should inspire confidence and optimism. (Believe me, you'll know when this is the case and when it isn't.) Your wife deserves a doctor who takes time to answer her questions, without seeming impatient or condescending. And she certainly doesn't want a doctor who pressures her with misleading or inappropriate comments. Such as? If a doctor discourages you from getting a second opinion, for instance, that's a good reason to get one. Here are five other dubious declarations, drawn from my wife's experience and from experiences that other women have had as they tried to make a decision about surgery.

#1. After a biopsy, cancer cells spread rapidly. You have to make up your mind about your surgery right away. "That's nonsense, and we've known that for years," says Dr. Alley. "That guy's an idiot." But that's what a Florida surgeon told Mary Anne Jacobsen, as he urged her to have a mastectomy. As she remembers it, the doctor said the cancer was spreading very quickly "because of the wire biopsy" and "a radical mastectomy had to be done as soon as possible." She asked about seeking a second opinion at an academic center, and the doctor said, "That'll take too long and you need to get it done, and get it done now."

Mary Anne and her husband, Rich, did pursue a second opinion, from a breast specialist at the Mayo Clinic in Jacksonville, and she's glad she did. The doc thought a lumpectomy was appropriate, and that's what Mary Anne chose. "Anyone who rushes you into a decision is suspect," says Dr. Drogula. "Breast cancer is a serious medical condition and shouldn't be ignored, but you usually have a month from diagnosis before anything changes." (The exception would be if your wife has inflammatory or especially aggressive breast cancer.)

#2. I'd recommend a mastectomy because you won't be happy with the cosmetic outcome of a lumpectomy. That's what a surgeon at our HMO told my wife. He explained that the tumor was so close to Marsha's nipple that the appearance of her breast wouldn't be pleasing after a lumpectomy. Such a statement could be valid. It could also be the opinion of a doctor who is not skillful at lumpectomies or who doesn't fully understand that many women would like very much to keep a breast if they can. Marsha sought a second opinion from a surgeon who did not work for the HMO. ("It's on your own nickel," the HMO surgeon said, although "your own $150" would be more like it.)

It was money well spent. "Breasts are very forgiving," Dr. Drogula said, endorsing lumpectomy plus radiation as a viable treatment. She told my wife there would be a little dent in her breast. But that was a choice for Marsha to make: a breast with a dent, or no breast at all.

#3. If you have a lumpectomy followed by radiation, the radiation will change the breast's architecture, and future cancers will be hard to spot. "Another garbage reason" for a mastectomy, says Dr. Alley. "Don't you want to go back to these guys and say, 'Where are you coming from?'"

I sure do, because that's another misstatement that a surgeon made to my wife.

By contrast, here's what our radiation oncologist told us: After radiation, the breast cancer patient has a baseline mammogram. Then the monitoring begins. Some women might have lumpy, dense breasts that are difficult to check for tumors, or breasts that have many suspicious calcifications that will make it difficult to notice any future tumor. Those conditions might argue for a mastectomy. But the surgeon shouldn't blame radiation, and your wife shouldn't take the surgeon's word for it. Encourage her to talk to her radiologist (the mammogram reader) as well and her radiation oncologist (who administers the radiation) before making a decision.

#4. I can tell you'll always worry about a recurrence if you have a lumpectomy, so mastectomy is what I'd recommend. Unless the surgeon can read your wife's mind, she shouldn't be swayed by second-guessing. "A woman is vulnerable at this point, and she's going to be more subject to believing the doctor who says, 'You need a mastectomy, because I can tell you're going to worry about recurrence,'" Dr. Alley says. "Whereas the husband can be a little more objective and say, 'Wait a minute, this doctor just met you 5 minutes ago. How does he know what you're going to be thinking a year from now?'"

#5. If this were my wife, this is what I would recommend. Doctors mean well when they make this kind of declaration. Husbands love it: "Wow, he's telling me the secret standard of care for doctor's wives!" Women like it, too. "I'm often asked, 'If I were your wife, what would you tell me?'" says Dr. Tsangaris. His answer: "I know what my wife would choose, but you are not my wife. You need to choose the treatment you are most comfortable with." Besides, doctors concede that they're notoriously bad at caring for family members. This rule applies for female surgeons, too. When a patient asks Susan Love, M.D., breast surgeon and chairman of the board of the Susan Love Research Foundation in Los Angeles, what she would do if she were in the patient's place, Dr. Love replies that she's not in the patient's place, and she doesn't know what she'd do if she were to face breast cancer.

THE CHOICE IS HERS

Remember, you're the sounding board, not the chairman of the board. Your wife may be torn between a lumpectomy and a mastectomy. She may find that a mastectomy affords her greater peace of mind, even if lumpectomy is considered a viable treatment. "Women are more willing to embark on mastectomy as a choice than men are to recommend it," says Dr. Drogula. "Husbands don't want to sound like they're saying, 'Cut off my wife's breast.'"

Besides, she's probably not going to listen to you. After all, it's her breast, and her life. "My wife developed breast cancer when she was 41, about 12 years ago," says Dr. Fred Smith. "I was a spouse, and also an oncologist." But his cancer expertise did not give him special clout. "She wanted a mastectomy. I thought she would be a perfectly good candidate for lumpectomy and radiation." That's the message he heard from the surgeon and radiation oncologist they saw as well. "You could hear the bias toward breast preservation," he says. "But she kept going back to mastectomy. She asked me, 'What should I do?'

"The point is," he told her, "I don't know what you should do." His wife knew what was right for her—a mastectomy. And reserving his judgment was the right thing for him to do.

TIPS ➢➢➢

1. "You want someone seeing breast cancer cases every week," says breast surgeon Cynthia Drogula, M.D., who practices in Washington, D.C. And you want to know what the doctor is doing to keep up with breast cancer—is he or she going to conferences and meetings?
2. For a breast specialist, sentinel node biopsy should be the standard of care. That's the removal of one or two lymph nodes—the first ones that cancer would be likely to reach—to check for cancerous cells. Additional nodes are removed only if the sentinel nodes test positive.
3. Not every surgeon is an advocate of lumpectomy. In fact, the rates of the breast-conserving lumpectomy (over mastectomy) are higher on the coasts and in big cities. For peace of mind, patients living in other areas—or any patient who goes to a general surgeon who does not see a lot of breast cancer patients—may want to seek a second opinion from a breast specialist.

➢ BONUS TIP

If your wife's surgeon talks about a "lesion," that's just a less-charged term for the tumor. A lesion is an area of abnormality in the breast. It can be cancerous—although not all lesions are. I don't know about you, but I liked using the word "lesion"—it wasn't quite as upsetting as "tumor" or "lump."

PARSING THE PATHOLOGY REPORT

After your wife's surgery, the hospital's pathology department examines the tumor and prepares a report. Her cancer docs get a copy. So does your wife. And she should be able to discern certain key facts among semi-mysterious terms like "non-neoplastic breast tissue" and "inferomedial."

Stage. The pathology report will determine your wife's cancer stage (stages are explained on page 118). "Stage trumps everything else," says Bill Smith, M.D., chairman of the department of pathology at Suburban Hospital in Bethesda, Maryland. The staging guides the oncologist and radiation oncologist as they determine the appropriate chemotherapy and radiation treatments.

Tumor size. Stated in centimeters. Bigger is typically worse, although the tumor's rate of growth is also important to weigh, particularly for smaller tumors, if the doctor is trying to make a decision about the need for chemotherapy.

Grade. The aggressiveness of the tumor is scored, from I to III. As in golf, the lower the score, the better.

Margins. When a lumpectomy is performed, the report will tell how close the tumor was to the margins—a number like 0.2 centimeters. The goal is to have clear margins, which means the entire tumor was removed and no cancer remains. If margins are not clear, or are too close to the tumor for the surgeon's comfort, the surgeon can operate again to remove any cancerous tissue that remains in the breast (or a mastectomy might be recommended). There's not universal accord on margins. Different doctors and hospitals might be satisfied with as little as 1 millimeter or might want as much as 1 centimeter.

Lymph nodes. The report will state how many lymph nodes were sampled and whether they tested positive or negative for cancer.

Hormone receptors. If your wife's tumor is estrogen receptor-positive and/or progesterone receptor-positive, she is a candidate for hormonal therapy—an estrogen-blocking drug like tamoxifen that cuts the risk of a local recurrence. The "percent positive" may or may not be stated in the report. Even a weak positive of 1 percent can qualify a patient for hormonal therapies, says Dr. Smith. If the percentage isn't given, ask about it.

If your wife can't find any one of these six points on her pathology report, she should go over the report with her doctor. In certain cases—for example, if there's an unusual finding—the surgeon, oncologist, or radiation oncologist might want a second reading at another lab.

What if your wife would like a second reading, because, well, it makes her more comfortable? The cost of peace of mind isn't too high—about $100 to $200, says Dr. Smith. Nor does it take a lot of effort—the lab pops the slides in a Fed Ex envelope and off they go. Your wife can ask her oncologist, or the lab that did the first report, to recommend a lab that works regularly with breast tumors.

If your wife is seeking a second opinion from doctors at another institution, that's a logical place to turn for a second pathology reading. The oncologist will probably want the in-house pathologist to file a report anyway, so your wife will be speeding up the process by sending her slides ahead.

Your Pre-Op Instructions

What to expect in the hospital

Your wife will get precise instructions about her surgery—which tests she needs to have done, what time she should stop eating and drinking the night before, when to arrive at the hospital.

I'm going to assume you're coming along for the surgery. Actually, I'm going to tell you: *come along for the surgery.* Instead of being fearful, be positive. "It's transformation surgery," Al Shockney told his wife, Lillie. Out comes the cancerous tumor, and, as Lillie puts it, your wife's survival odds "sail up the chart."

Progressive hospitals set up a pre-op visit that includes the husband, but many spouses aren't that lucky. If you're among the uninitiated, here are your marching orders.

Arrival time. Your wife checks in, changes into the never-fashionable hospital gown and slippers, and is prepped for surgery—IVs for hydration and anesthesia, for example. You can stay with her most of the time, except perhaps when she's undressing. If her veins are small or "difficult" to tap, you or she should ask for the best person to start the IV—a skilled nurse or an adept anesthesiologist. Using a butterfly needle (shaped like its namesake, it is smaller than a regular needle) might help. This is a good time for the wedding ring handoff. You can wear it (if it fits) or hold it in a safe spot until after the surgery. (In some cases, the hospital staff will let the ring stay on but cover it with tape.) Eyeglasses and false teeth can be entrusted to you or to a nurse, who will return them to your wife in the recovery room.

The waiting game, round 1. There she is, all dressed down and nowhere to go; that is, until a staff member arrives to wheel her from her curtained cubicle to the O.R. Stay by her side. If conversation is difficult, just reach out and touch her. For some couples, the antiseptic, impersonal pre-op room might discourage physical contact. I watched one husband and wife whiling away the minutes before the wife's lumpectomy. She was propped up in bed, hooked up to an IV. Her loyal spouse sat silently in a chair by her side. It looked as if they wanted to connect in a physical way but weren't sure how. Finally, the woman plopped her slippered feet into her husband's lap. "It's a lot warmer there," she quipped. A smile spread across his worried face, and he began massaging her toes.

Pre-op rituals. I didn't have any, other than to kiss my wife and tell her that I loved her. But some guys (and their wives) are quite creative.

Dorothy Davis had her husband, John, family members, and the minister from her church on hand at the hospital before her mastectomy. "We said all kinds of prayers for the doctors and nurses," says Dorothy, "and before I went into surgery I was anointed with oil by the reverend."

Then there's the inspirational story I heard from clinical therapist and cancer specialist Lora Matz. When Matz was working at the Virginia Piper Cancer Institute at Minneapolis's Abbott Northwestern Hospital, a 30-ish husband came to see her the night before his wife's double mastectomy. The man confessed that he'd been a workaholic and a neglectful spouse, and wanted to make amends. Matz put him through a relaxation exercise and told him to contact his "wife guide" (you know, the spirit that tells you what to buy for your beloved on her birthday) to see what to do. And eureka, he got it! He rushed out to a jewelry store, bought two ID bracelets, and had them engraved on the spot, one with his name, one with his wife's. (Try a mall shop or a department store, Matz suggests.)

He unveiled the bracelets at the hospital before surgery, and told his wife he'd wear the one with her name, and she should wear the one with his. He said, "I'll be there, standing by your side and stroking your head."

GUY TALK

"I stayed with Tricia until she went in for surgery, cracking up about how doped up she was. Waiting room anxiety is always going to be one of those things that overwhelms us. The way to avoid the anxiety is to watch TV, read, get lost in the moment. I seldom talked to people. I went into my own world, my inner protection."

—DAVE COMO, 35
Pittsburgh

Most hospitals won't let a patient wear jewelry in the operating room—partly to prevent anything from disappearing and partly because metal objects can increase the risk of shock. Perhaps the staff removed her bracelet during the surgery. But the point of the story isn't as much the bracelet as the sentiment behind it.

Be prepared to cry. The last glimpse of your wife as she is wheeled off—or walked in—to surgery might bring on tears. "It is difficult to put into words the helplessness I felt as Laurie was taken into the operating room," says Jim Finkelstein, whose wife underwent a bilateral mastectomy. "This is the woman I married, who birthed our children, and built the home we know," says David Houser, 52, of his wife, Conny. "You want to jump in her place and say, 'Do the surgery on me.'"

The waiting game, round 2. Welcome to the waiting room. I hope you enjoy your stay. Maybe you'll be alone. Maybe you'll have a few support people of your own—your in-laws, your parents, other family members or friends. The big question is: How long do you have to wait? When the surgeon meets your wife to go over the consent form, ask for an estimate. (It probably will be about 2 hours until the surgeon comes to report on how things went—maybe a little less, maybe a little more.) And ask where the surgeon will come to find you. You sure don't want to be in the wrong waiting area. Some hospitals lend a beeper to the husband; he'll get a 2-minute warning before the surgeon's arrival, so he's free to roam to the cafeteria, or go to the bathroom, or perhaps even take a short walk outside instead of being a waiting-room prisoner.

What to bring. Stuff to pass the time. A laptop, a book, papers from work. A music headset might be a nice distraction. David Freeman, 40, of

Rochester, New York, brought a book on nautical knots and some rope to the hospital when his wife, Yosepha, underwent a bilateral mastectomy and reconstruction. "I tied knots while I sat there," he says. That might draw some stares, but it's definitely better than sitting and feeling as if *you're* all tied up in knots.

Phone info. Hospitals typically ban cell phones in areas where monitoring devices are in use—the recovery room, patient rooms. They may be banned in waiting rooms, too. Bring coins for a pay phone, or a calling card, and a list of phone numbers of people you'll want to call. You can also walk outside the building to use your cell or find an area of the hospital where cell phones are allowed.

Food. Your call: Bring a sandwich from home, or pick up something at the hospital cafeteria. My fear was that I'd be out of the waiting room when the doctor came looking, so I erred on the side of caution and packed snacks.

TV tip. If there's a TV in the waiting room, whatever show is on will be imprinted upon your memory banks as "the cancer show." I still cringe whenever *The Price Is Right* comes on. And you might not be able to change the channel or turn the infernal thing off. "I was ready to bring in wire cutters," says Allen Salzberg, 50, of Queens, New York. I know I don't need to say this, but that's definitely a bad idea.

The waiting game, round 3. After the surgery is over, the surgeon will brief you on how it went. Ask how long you'll have to wait before you can reunite with your wife in the recovery room. It'll probably be about an hour. When 90 minutes had passed since the surgery ended, I checked with the volunteer manning the desk in the waiting room. You might be feeling impatient. But you'll get a better response if you simply state the facts. Kyle Terrell, a surgical oncology nurse practitioner at the Johns Hopkins Breast Center in Baltimore, suggests saying something like, "My wife finished surgery an hour ago. I'm wondering how she's doing and when I can see her." Maybe the answer will be that the hospital was hit by four admissions and things are running slowly. Or maybe your wife hasn't awakened yet from the anesthesia.

The right way to get attention. The nurses in the recovery room were extraordinarily kind and helpful to my wife and to me. All I had to do was ask for help, and they'd do their best, even if it was to bring a ginger ale for Marsha to sip.

The wrong way to get attention. There may be a moment when you feel as if you're ready to explode because you think the staff is neglecting your wife. Ted Tsangaris, M.D., the Hopkins breast surgeon, remembers a very supportive husband whose wife had a mastectomy followed by reconstruction. After the lengthy and arduous surgery, she was in pain and the pain medication wasn't working. The husband "had a meltdown," Dr. Tsangaris says. "He turned into this unpleasant, surly guy, writing everyone's name down and acting out. It was obvious he had lost control. He felt helpless and felt that the only way he could help was to stir the pot and yell and scream at all the health-care providers." That's not a recommended course of action.

But, Dr. Tsangaris concedes, "It got my attention. I made the change in pain medicine."

A wiser choice might be to have a pad and pen with you, and to start taking notes about how long it takes for a response to be met. If need be, visit the nurse's station and ask to speak to a supervisor.

A job for you. If your wife had a mastectomy or an axillary dissection—lymph nodes removed from her armpit—she may have to stay overnight. In the latter case, she should not have her blood pressure or blood draws taken on the side of the dissection—that could bring on lymphedema, or swelling of the arm. My good friend (and breast cancer survivor) Katy Kelly told me, "Ask the nurses to make a big sign not to do any work on the axillary dissection side." I thought she was maybe a little overzealous. But the first nurse who came into Marsha's room went straight for the right arm. I asked the nurse for paper and a magic marker, and made a big bold sign to post on the bulletin board over the bed. I wasn't happy about the lack of communication in the hospital. But I don't have to tell you that, as a guy, I was thrilled to feel as if I had actually fixed something. (Keep in mind that this isn't a one-time problem. Your wife should *never* have blood pressure cuffs or needle sticks on the affected arm because of the ongoing risk of lymphedema. See the chapter The New Normal on page 272 for more information.)

P.S. She might come home with a drain. If your wife has had a mastectomy and/or an axillary dissection, she will come out of surgery with a bulbous plastic drain or two hanging from a long strip of tubing. An armpit drain siphons off lymphatic fluid that would otherwise build up in the armpit. The mastectomy drain handles fluid that would otherwise fill the surgical cavity. Periodically, the drains must be emptied.

Your wife won't be happy about any of this. "Women hate drains," says Cynthia Drogula, M.D., a Washington, D.C., breast surgeon. "Oh God, they hate drains."

To make matters worse, sometimes the tube that leads to the drain will become clogged.

At the hospital, the surgeon or a nurse practitioner will give you specific instructions on how to empty the drain. They should also show you and your wife what to do in case of a clog in the tube, using your finger and a pen. Don't panic. My medical skills consist of removing splinters, and it really wasn't too hard to unclog the drain.

Dr. Drogula says half the husbands she sees are happy to be drain managers, half aren't. "Some look at me like I'm nuts if I suggest that they give a hand. Others are all into it."

If neither you nor your wife is comfortable being on drain duty, then you need to arrange for a visiting nurse before leaving the hospital.

Eventually, the fluid begins diminishing. When the 24-hour total is less than 30 cc's—that's the equivalent of about 2 tablespoons—out comes the drain. Often, it only takes a week, but it can take longer—up to a month in some cases. The removal of the drain is obviously a good step—a sign that your wife's body is returning to normal. But it also means your wife is ready for the next stage of her treatment. And if the next stage is chemo, you may find yourself pining for the days when the biggest headache was drain maintenance.

Missing a Breast

The impact of a mastectomy

She still remembers the look. It was the first time he saw her chest after she came home from the hospital, minus one breast. She was standing in the bathroom, getting undressed. Walking by, he caught a glimpse of what she calls, with sardonic humor, "the remains of the day." And she caught a look—"a flicker of distaste across his face." A "micro-expression" that lasted mere seconds, but an expression that she has never forgotten.

She knows that her chest was not a pretty sight. There was swelling and redness from the incision and the stitches. She had not had reconstructive surgery.

She never said anything to him. He never said anything to her.

He was her long-term, live-in boyfriend, who had stood by her during diagnosis and treatment, braving a blizzard to drive her to the hospital for her mastectomy and bringing her parents in from the airport to her home. In other words, he was more of a husband than some till-death-do-us-part husbands. But then came the look. The look was, as it turns out, a harbinger of bad things to come. Three years later, he did "the grand dump," as she puts it, and he gave her the impression that he would have walked out long before, only he couldn't just leave her right after she had been diagnosed with cancer. She can't quite believe he was really ready to say goodbye at that time. Not when she remembers how he hugged her when she was afraid, and how much that meant to her.

A few more years have gone by. She is healthy, and she looks good. She has moved on with her life. But looking back, she wonders: *What if?* What if, on that day of unexpected revelation, she had said to him, "What was that look for?" or "It doesn't look too good to me, either." Instead, she was silent; and even now, she is haunted by the bitter memory of the look—and by the unspoken words that might have saved their relationship.

So, dear husband, don't let your stare do the talking for you. Especially in the aftermath of a mastectomy.

FIRST REACTIONS

"Breasts are a big deal in America," says TV journalist Linda Ellerbee, who had a double mastectomy 12 years ago. "Just look around you."

The loss of a breast is a big deal, too. But there's no way to predict how your wife will react to the loss of a defining female part. Each year, about 101,000 women undergo a mastectomy, and I'd venture to say there are 101,000 different ways that the surgery plays out. So a breast cancer husband has to be ready for anything. You may feel as if you are walking a tightrope over a pit of eggshells. Say the wrong thing (or say nothing at all), cast a judgmental glance . . . and watch out.

The very thought of a mastectomy is enough to plunge some women into a wordless depression. That's what happened to my wife after we visited a surgeon who recommended a bilateral mastectomy. Marsha was cloaked in a raw and impenetrable sorrow. She retreated into herself. Nothing I said made a difference. I told her I loved her and not her breasts. She lashed out at me, "How would you feel if a doctor wanted to cut off your penis?"

My hands involuntarily traveled to cup my boys. And my wife wondered what to do about her girls, who had presented breast-cancer false alarms over the years, and now had betrayed her, as it were, by developing the real thing.

Needless to say, my wife's comments made me feel awful. After all, I was just trying to share what was in my heart. When I interviewed psychologist

Anne Coscarelli, Ph.D, I asked her if I'd done something wrong. Her answer was, "No." It's important to express such feelings, says Dr. Coscarelli, who directs the UCLA Ted Mann Family Resource Center at the Jonsson Comprehensive Cancer Center in Los Angeles. She sees a lot of breast cancer husbands—not all of them, but a significant number—who tell their wives, "I don't care whether you have breasts or not. It's not your breasts I care about. I care about losing you. I love you and I want you in my life. That's the most important thing to me." But husbands need to understand that even such loving sentiments might not blunt the initial explosion of psychic pain. Many months later, I asked Marsha what I could have said or done to make a difference when she was feeling so blue. Her answer: "Nothing." She didn't want to hear, "There, there," or "It's not so bad."

She was grateful that I was by her side and that I hugged her and told her I loved her. "But even then, I still had to go through it," she says of her sorrow at the prospect of losing both breasts.

And I realized I was guilty of the crime of being a husband who wanted to fix things, to say the magic words that would banish Marsha's depression, when what I needed to do was to shut up and let her mourn the potential loss of her breasts.

WEIGHING THE FACTS

The day after Marsha made that cutting remark about my manhood, we saw a breast specialist who felt that the first surgeon's recommendation, based on a desire to remove any fear of recurrence, was not my wife's only option. The breast specialist explained that Marsha was a good candidate for breast conservation, meaning lumpectomy instead of mastectomy. The less severe surgery would most likely be able to remove the tumor. In addition, the surgeon told us that a lumpectomy followed by radiation treatments yields a rate of local recurrence—that is, in the breast itself—just a few percentage points higher than the rate for mastectomy patients. Then we saw another breast specialist who was of the same opinion. I probably don't have to tell you which surgical option Marsha chose. When she asked me, "What do you think?" I choked back a few tears and said, "Lumpectomy sounds good to me."

Like Marsha, many women with early-stage breast cancer have a choice between lumpectomy and mastectomy. And it's not a life-or-death decision. Over the years, studies have shown that the long-term survival rate for women with breast cancer stages 0 through II is the same whether the surgery is lumpectomy or mastectomy. The lumpectomy patients, however, have a 40 percent chance of a local recurrence—another cancer in the same breast—unless they have radiation following their surgery. With a lumpectomy *plus* radiation, the patient has about a 10 percent chance of local recurrence for invasive cancer.

Meanwhile, even with a mastectomy, an early-stage cancer patient runs a small risk of local recurrence—as low as 1 percent in some cases, but typically in the 5 to 10 percent range. That's one of the many subtle points about breast cancer that patients (and their husbands) sometimes miss. It defies logic—remove the breast and remove the chances of a second tumor in that breast, right? Not quite. A new cancer can grow along the skin or the chest wall, where the breast formerly sat. The risk of recurrence for mastectomy patients is higher if the tumor is 5 centimeters or larger and has spread to four or more lymph nodes, or if the patient has inflammatory breast cancer.

Breast surgeon Susan Love, M.D., in her eponymous *Dr. Susan Love's Breast Book,* tells of a woman who had a small tumor but opted for a bilateral mastectomy "because she never wanted to deal with it again." But she did have to deal with it again. A year later, the cancer recurred in her scar. The woman was furious; she said that no doctor had ever mentioned that such a thing could occur.

Like this woman, some breast cancer patients have a choice between lumpectomy and mastectomy and opt for the more radical surgery. Three years ago, Lois Hazel learned that she had a 2.5-centimeter tumor and one positive lymph node. The surgeon presented the two options: lumpectomy or mastectomy. Lois wanted a mastectomy: "I just wanted to be as aggressive as I could." And that was okay with her husband, Dale. "Listen, I'm madly in love with this woman," he says. "I don't care if she's got one breast or two or six." And Lois, who was 56 when she was diagnosed, looked at it from a practical standpoint. "I had nursed my babies. That's what my breasts were there for. I didn't feel it was going to change who I am."

MAKING A DECISION

One of breast cancer's most appalling ironies is that a mastectomy may be the surgery of choice for a woman with no cancer at all. It happened to a friend of mine as I was writing this book. She e-mailed me that a mammogram had revealed pre-cancerous cells in both breasts. She didn't have cancer—yet. But she was very likely to develop cancer. The only way to prevent it was to remove her breasts, since there wasn't a cancerous lump, just those scattered cells. So that's what she did.

TV journalist Linda Ellerbee found herself in a similar dilemma after her diagnosis. There was a large cancerous lump in her left breast, and there were precancerous cells and microcalcifications in the right. Ellerbee's surgeon, the illustrious Dr. Love, told her that she could undergo a left breast mastectomy and keep an eye on the other breast. Or she could schedule a bilateral mastectomy. Ellerbee opted for the latter: "The main reason is that I did not want to lie awake at night wondering when that precancerous condition would turn into a cancerous condition. The other reason is that I had very large breasts, and if I lost one I could never match it. Take my breast, save my life! To hell with my breasts! That was a decision I've never regretted."

Or your wife may be one of the women who schedules a mastectomy with nary a precancerous cell in evidence. If a woman has a family history of breast cancer—her mom, her sister, or her grandmother had the disease—she herself could carry a gene that puts her at a high risk of developing breast cancer. She can take a blood test to see if she carries one of the breast cancer genes that scientists have identified. If the test is positive and she has had no cancers, she can lower her risk substantially by undergoing a bilateral mastectomy.

No matter what your wife's situation, she will weigh the facts and her fears. She will talk to her doctor, and perhaps seek second and third and even fourth opinions. Throughout this process, your role is to support her as she makes a decision that is based on sound medical information, a decision that diminishes her anxiety, a decision that will let her move on with her life instead of feeling paralyzed by the fear of cancer. You can ask her questions: How would you feel if you didn't have a mastectomy and later had a second cancer and then had to face a mastectomy? How would you feel if you delayed the removal of a cancer-free breast to make sure you really want to go ahead with it?

You also could propose doing what breast surgeon Ted Tsangaris, M.D., of the Johns Hopkins Breast Center in Baltimore, recommends for a patient who has the option of a lumpectomy or mastectomy, but is leaning toward the latter—perhaps because she mistakenly believes it'll take care of her cancer forever. He suggests visiting a plastic surgeon to find out what reconstruction entails—a lot of surgery and recuperative time as well. Some of these women come back to Dr. Tsangaris and say, "I don't want the lumpectomy; I feel comfortable with the mastectomy." Others come back eager to preserve their breast.

In the end, your wife has to come up with the answer that's right for her.

IN THE OPERATING ROOM

A mastectomy itself is fairly simple and straightforward—actually a bit less complicated than a lumpectomy, which involves a series of subtle excisions: first for the tumor, then for surrounding tissue to ensure that the margins are clear, meaning that no cancer is left behind. And a mastectomy is not nearly as brutal as it was back in 1904 when it was first devised as a breast cancer treatment. The original total radical mastectomy was quite disfiguring; the surgeon removed all the chest wall muscles and exposed the rib cage, based on the (erroneous) principle that taking more tissue would lower the risk of recurrent disease.

I watched a modern-day mastectomy at Johns Hopkins University Hospital. The patient was draped with blue sheets, so only her torso was visible. The surgeon had drawn a blue circle around her right breast. Working methodically with a styluslike instrument called a Bovie—a combination cutter and cauterizer—a seasoned doctor and a young resident severed the mammary gland. In 59 minutes, they were done. I couldn't help but comment on how little time the surgery took. The surgeon said it would have gone even faster if he hadn't been working with a resident. The transformation was startling. One minute this woman had a breast on her chest. Fifty-nine minutes later, her chest was flat, indistinguishable from a male torso, with a gap where the breast used to be. A nurse placed the breast itself—the circle of nippled skin and the mass of amber fat and scarlet blood vessels beneath—into a plastic bag. It was sent to the pathology department, where the tumor would be evaluated so the doctors could know more about the patient's prognosis.

So that is what goes on in the operating room, while you sweat it out in the waiting room, pacing and pondering.

SHAMPOO AND SOLACE

You will most certainly end up waiting longer than 59 minutes. More like a couple of hours, considering the time it takes from the moment they start the IV for anesthesia until the surgery is complete and they wheel your wife to the recovery room. The doctor should come and speak with you in the waiting room after the surgery to tell you how things went. I remember worrying that I'd somehow be forgotten, because breast cancer husbands don't get a lot of attention. I guess I worry too much. The first thing the surgeon at Hopkins said after the mastectomy was done: "I'm going to go tell her significant other how things went."

After the doctor speaks with you, you'll have a little more waiting to do, maybe an hour or so, until your wife has shaken off a bit of the anesthesia and is ready for your company. Or maybe less. "Coming out of surgery, they expected her to be out for 2 hours," says Dave Como of his wife's bilateral mastectomy and reconstructive surgery. "Within half an hour, Trish was up, going, 'I'm hungry. I want a hamburger. And how do they look?'" ("They" were her reconstructed breasts. And, Como says, they looked pretty good.)

Assuming there are no complications from a mastectomy, your wife should go home that night or the next day, with a soft surgical bra that contains a temporary breast form. She will have a drain or two hanging from the wound to drain off lymphatic fluid that results from the removal of breast tissue, and a drain hanging from her armpit if an axillary dissection was needed. Drains must be emptied several times a day for those first few days. This is something you can help out with, if you're a hands-on kind of guy. A nurse should instruct you on how to do this before sending your wife home from the hospital.

Your wife will be fatigued, and sore in the chest area. She will have lost some range of motion on the mastectomy side, so raising her arm above her head may prove difficult (although exercises can help her regain her flexibility). She can shower after 2 days, with her drains in place, but she might need some help washing her hair. One option is for her to stand with her head over the kitchen sink while you serve as shampoo boy, but it's hardly much fun for her.

One clever husband brought a lawn chair into his oversize shower stall. Linda Anderson, age 58, of Minneapolis, knelt over the side of the tub, with pillows and towels cushioning her mastectomy scars, while husband Allen washed. "I was trying to explain how to wash my hair. It was like teaching somebody how to walk," Linda laughs. "She seemed so delicate, I didn't want to do anything that would cause too much pain," Allen says.

Any tips? "They really want their scalps massaged," Allen laughs. For further instruction, watch Robert Redford shampoo Meryl Streep's hair in *Out of Africa*.

RECOVERY TIME

It will probably take a couple of weeks before your wife feels like herself again, although different women recover at different rates. "Husbands should realize there's a certain amount of grieving for your lost body," says novelist Carol Shields, recalling her mastectomy. "I'm not sure whether men think of that automatically—what it's like to lose a vital part of yourself."

The physical recovery might be less traumatic than the psychological adjustment. "Pain-wise, that was a piece of cake," says Lois Hazel of her mastectomy. "The axillary dissection [that is, the removal of lymph nodes from her armpit] was much worse." Nonetheless, your wife most likely won't be able to lift heavy objects, cook, grocery shop, or do laundry for a couple of weeks after the surgery. The doctor will give her a list of restrictions. And you know what that means—you're the designated pinch hitter.

You can help your wife rebuild her strength. Jack Ennis, 53, of Hampton, Virginia, began taking his wife, Nancy, on daily walks just 4 days after her mastectomy. They covered 2 miles the first time, which was a bit much. But they kept on walking together on a daily basis. "We felt if you act sick and

---

MEN WITH MASTECTOMIES

If you're worried that your wife is doing too much after her surgery, try to put yourself in her place before you panic. Actually, you don't have to. I can tell you exactly how a guy might react.

Each year, about 1,600 men in the United States are diagnosed with breast cancer. I interviewed three men who had been diagnosed and treated. Each of them had a mastectomy. The surgery is not as devastating for a man's self-image, although as 52-year-old Herb Palm of Easton, Maryland, jokes, "I'll never look like Arnold Schwarzenegger." (He's quick to add that there's no disfigurement and his scar is virtually unnoticeable.) In my very small sample, two of the three men went out and mowed the lawn, drains and all, as soon as they got home from the hospital. I asked why. "I got up on my tractor and mowed the grass all day to take my mind off the breast cancer," Herb said. "It needed mowing," said Mark Goldstein, 71, of Randolph, New Jersey, who had a mastectomy 15 years ago. He used a push mower on his overgrown grass and calls the mowing his "first act of defiance toward the disease."

Ya gotta love guys.

My point isn't that you should encourage your wife to mow the lawn. But rather, you should realize that after a significant surgery like a mastectomy, a patient needs to reassert a sense of identity: They're still the same people they were just 24 hours before. Mark Goldstein's family came up with a clever way to make sure Mark got the message. He loved to scuba dive, so his wife and kids bought a scuba-diver action figure and placed it by his bedside in the hospital. "Because I had put off a scuba diving trip for the operation," he says, "they were reminding me I should pick up my life after breast cancer."

Within the year, he was under the water again.

And if you think your wife should forget about her breast cancer once treatment is over, take a lesson from Mark. He has gone on to run more than 135 Komen Races for the Cure.

act like a patient, you'll probably be sick and be a patient longer," he says. He brought a jogging suit to the hospital for his wife so she wouldn't languish in nightgowns, and he made sure it zipped up the front for ease of donning and doffing.

Some women don't want to wait 4 days before getting back on the treadmill—literally. Kyle Terrell, the nurse practitioner at Johns Hopkins, recalls a call from a frantic husband the day after a mastectomy surgery. His wife was on their home treadmill, ready to trek a couple of miles.

"I talked to her and she was fine," Terrell says. A patient who is not yet steady on her feet shouldn't be treadmilling, but this woman was doing okay. She got up, ate breakfast, and began her workout as she did every morning.

THE UNVEILING

Some couples sail into their post-mastectomy life with no qualms. For others, the voyage isn't smooth.

The husband may be afraid to look. "Try to focus on the person and not the malady," says Jack Ennis. "The person you fell in love with and interact with is certainly not a breast."

Or the woman may be reluctant to show her scarred chest to her husband. "I work with a lot of women who find themselves repulsive, so they feel they must be repulsive to others," says psychiatrist Mary Jane Massie, M.D., who practices at Memorial Sloan-Kettering in New York City. "So I say, if your husband had testicular cancer and had lost his hair and had a plastic replacement testicle, would that really disgust you? And they look at me like, well, no, that's my husband. Of course it wouldn't." If your wife has similar qualms, then you might take a deep breath and pose a similar question.

Lillie Shockney, the Johns Hopkins nurse and cancer survivor who seems as if nothing could intimidate her, was nervous at the thought of showing her husband what she looked like with one breast. She could not have reconstruction at the time because of a severe reaction to anesthesia. Her husband, Al, seems like a Rock of Gibraltar who wouldn't be fazed a bit by the sight.

GUY TALK

"She didn't show me for the longest of times. She felt she was ugly, deformed, scarred, that I was going to be repulsed. I said, 'Absolutely not.' It didn't repulse me at all. I said, 'I don't care. You're here, that's what matters.'"

—ERIC LUDWICK, 55
Montreal, whose wife, Annette, had a bilateral mastectomy—and eventually chose to have reconstructive surgery

Yet there was this conspiracy of silence. Lillie hadn't set a date for the premiere, and Al didn't know what to do about it.

Lillie's surgeon asked her about her plans to let Al see the wound. She told the surgeon she thought she'd let a few days go by. Her surgeon went, "Hmm." And Lillie learned an important lesson. When your surgeon goes "Hmm," watch out.

The day she was to go home from the hospital, Al was supposed to pick her up at 9:00 A.M. But at 6:00 A.M., in he strode. "I couldn't sleep, babe," white-haired Al told his puckish, buxom bride. Then in came the surgeon. And off came the dressings. And Al saw the scar, and it was fine, and instead of wondering when she'd have the courage to show Al her breastless chest, Lillie could go home blissfully reassured that her dear husband loved her as she now was. And when they embraced, he told her, "Our hearts almost touched."

Now, you've got to know your wife and have a gut feeling for what her reaction might be. Some women would definitely not appreciate being blindsided by a husband. And some women are never really okay with showing a scarred chest to their partner. Venus Masselam, Ph.D., a psychologist who practices in Bethesda, Maryland, told me of a woman in her 70s who felt that way. "Think of the era in which she grew up," Dr. Masselam says. "There was a difference in how a woman's body was treated. And her husband did a good job. He respected her wishes. He didn't feel like he was shut out. He supported her in the effort. In other words, he was in on it with her. It wasn't like it was her thing, and she was cutting herself off from him. He was saying,

'I don't want to do anything that makes you feel uncomfortable.' That's the basis of understanding—and of tenderness."

GETTING REACQUAINTED

Other couples would like to return to an intimacy free of garments, but the hospital doesn't provide a road map.

Perhaps you'll have an easy adjustment. A well-done mastectomy incision is not scary to behold, says Lillie Shockney. Your wife will have "a smooth, flat chest, as if she were 10 years old again."

But it's perfectly natural to be nervous, says Ronnie Kaye, who had the surgery herself and has written about the experience in *Spinning Straw into Gold: Your Emotional Recovery from Breast Cancer.* As a psychotherapist in Marina del Rey, California, Kaye counsels other breast cancer patients on how to cope. She has advice for a nervous wife who wants to initiate post-mastectomy intimacy, and for a husband who has qualms about a first look.

There's nothing wrong with taking it slow. For starters, Kaye suggests that an apprehensive husband might want to look at a photograph of a woman who's had a mastectomy and no reconstruction. That way, Kaye explains, he can get used to the appearance of a woman who is missing a breast without running the risk of hurting his wife's feelings. "It takes away a lot of the pressure," she says. Post-surgery and post-divorce, Kaye showed a photograph of writer and breast cancer survivor Deena Metzger to a potential boyfriend. (Metzger's topless, post-mastectomy picture, with her arms outstretched and a tattoo of a tree branch concealing her scar, can be seen at www.deenametzger.com—just click on "tree poster" on the left-hand menu bar.) "He took a while to look at it and study it, and finally said, 'That's not bad.' After that, it was okay for us to get intimate."

You might also schedule a look at your wife's chest just to get reacquainted. Maybe the two of you can sit in, say, the living room when no one else is home. And the ground rules might be that your wife will take off her shirt and she'll not be wearing a bra. Then the two of you will have a "show-and-tell," Kaye suggests. You can talk about how the surgery has changed her appearance. Or maybe you'll just hug each other. But no sex allowed, Kaye says. "That's not the time for sex. It's unfair to ask a man to act sexually interested and maintain an erection in the face of shock or fear or ambivalence."

Then you may be ready for the next step. Ask your wife to take your hand and guide it and show you where it's fine to touch and where it's not. Or ask her a few questions: "Will anything I do hurt you or upset you?" Part of the problem may be that you're afraid to touch your wife's chest at all, lest you hurt her. Don't worry, she'll tell you if that happens.

And you can tell her what's in your heart. "I don't care what you're missing," one husband said to his wife. "That's not what you're about for me. I'm not counting how many of what you have. I just like being with you."

David Moyer told his wife, Brenda: "Your scar is beautiful, because it means you are going to live." As far as he's concerned, voluptuous breasts aren't essential for great sex. "If I want to see breasts, I can rent any movie in the video store, turn on the TV, open a magazine, or get on the Internet," he adds. "So what's the big deal about a breast?"

If you're the silent type, your wife might put you on the spot. Twenty-five years ago, Deborah Stewart, 50, of Bel Air, Maryland, flat out asked her husband: "Do you miss the breast?" She didn't know what he'd say, because he'd never said a word on the subject.

"I recall the question," says Don, 54, with the measured air of his profession—he's a CPA. "It's the last question I would have expected. I had to reflect, but it didn't take long. I just told her the truth." The truth was that yes, he did miss her breast. That made Deborah feel better, because she missed it, too.

TIPS >>>

1. Your wife may need time to mourn the loss of her breast. You can tell her how much you love her, and not her breasts, but this is not the time to play cheerleader.
2. You might want to visit a woman's boutique that carries garb for mastectomy patients. The store should sell camisoles that will hold your wife's post-surgery drains and will not rub on her incision.
3. Nervous about seeing your wife's scar? Looking at a picture of a woman with a mastectomy might help to prepare you. Type "mastectomy photograph" in an Internet search engine like Google.

> BONUS TIP

If your wife is looking for information on exercises to help her recover from a mastectomy, steer her to the Web site www.focusonhealing.org.

Booby Trap

As your wife weighs breast replacement options, just shut up and listen

Surreal.

That's the word that many breast cancer couples use to describe the process of seeking a replacement for a lost breast or breasts.

An estimated 60 percent of mastectomy patients decide they want reconstructive surgery—up from 40 percent a decade ago. If your wife is in this group, the two of you may find yourselves sitting in a plastic surgeon's office, leafing through a binder that holds before-and-after photos of nearly naked ladies. The pictures show only the torso—from just below the neck to just above the pubic hair line. The first shot shows a woman who is missing one or both breasts or is displaying her own natural breasts prior to a mastectomy. In the second, the woman has a brand-new breast or breasts (and maybe a flatter stomach, too, if the new breast was harvested from abdominal fat). "It's like some strange sort of pornography," says Larry Gold*, recalling his reaction when he and his newly diagnosed wife perused such a book.

Or, at some point, you may wind up shopping at a store that specializes in prostheses—that is, silicone-filled wedges that slip into specially built bras.

Cheryl Hoyt, who runs Cheryl's Health Boutique in Rockville, Maryland, recalls a husband who eyed one of the larger models and said to his wife, "You can be Dolly Parton right now!" He was kidding. I think.

FOLLOW HER LEAD

No one—including you—should tell your wife which choice to make. But that won't stop people from trying. At a breast cancer conference I attended, one woman stood and said she couldn't fathom why any mastectomy patient would not want to have reconstructive surgery. To which an indignant fellow survivor responded, "You have no right to make that judgment for the rest of us."

It's even worse when a husband exerts pressure. Lillie Shockney, the Johns Hopkins nurse and a breast cancer survivor, remembers a distressing case of one couple with two opinions. The wife wasn't ready to consider reconstruction. The husband was, and he wasn't shy about sharing his view. Lillie pulled this guy out of the doctor's office for a private chat, and asked, "How would you feel if your wife told you she wanted your penis to be bigger?"

I don't have to tell you what the husband replied.

But I do have to tell you what Lillie said next, "That's how you're making her feel when you tell her you want her to have reconstruction."

So what should the breast cancer husband do? "Shut up and listen," says Michael Olding, M.D., associate professor of surgery and chief of the Division of Plastic and Reconstructive Surgery at George Washington University. Now there's a phrase I've heard a time or 200 in the course of researching this book. If you need any more guidance, let me remind you of another excellent breast cancer husband motto, courtesy of Bobbye Sloan, breast cancer survivor and wife of Utah Jazz coach Jerry Sloan: "Follow her lead."

That doesn't mean you have to sit there nodding as if you're a bobblehead doll. "You can't be pushy, and you can't be a recluse," Bobbye elaborates. And then she repeats her words of wisdom, because we husbands sometimes need to be told what to do more than once: "You just follow her lead."

THE PROSTHESIS

As your wife considers her options, she may lead you to the nearest store that sells prosthetic devices. Some women want no part of another surgery or are not good candidates for reconstruction—they may have a history of heart or lung problems, smoking, or obesity. Women with late-stage breast cancer may be advised to delay reconstructive surgery. Or there may be other reasons they're not interested. "I didn't know if I would feel comfortable with something false," says Brenda Heil of Wausau, Wisconsin, who eventually had a bilateral mastectomy after breast cancer struck her at age 24.

A prosthesis can certainly create the illusion of a breast, but it is an imperfect solution. Your wife may, for example, feel that spontaneity has vanished. Whenever she wants to go out (or when friends stop by unexpectedly), she may feel she needs to pop in the prosthesis. Imagine if you had to stuff a sock in your briefs under the same circumstances, and you'll get the picture. She may also feel self-conscious exposing her one- or no-breasted chest, even to you. And if your wife forgets her breast replacement when she heads out to the office, you may find yourself, as one husband did, hurrying to her workplace with an unusual item to present to your unevenly chested spouse.

The prosthesis isn't a cheap fix. The price range for a prefab model is $250 to $500; the devices come in flesh or brown tones. A custom-made prosthesis might cost up to $3,000 (and can even be made with freckles and veins painted on to match your wife's skin). Just as medical insurance will cover reconstruction, it will cover the prosthesis—up to a point. Typically there's a $500 cap and no deductible on this item.

What's the difference between the lower- and higher-priced models? Think of it as Honda versus Lexus, the mavens say. At any price point, a prosthetic breast will get your wife where she's going, but an upper-end model will have a little more style. It'll feel more like breast tissue and less like rubber.

The other prosthetic option is a Perma-Form bra, which comes with one or two built-in foam prostheses (whichever your wife needs). The price is around $125, but your wife will need more than one of these bras, since they require three days to air dry after a spin in the washing machine. "A silicone prosthesis has a more natural feel," notes Lillie Shockney, who has tried both types. "The woman can feel as if her breast is really there." The Perma-Form bra, she reports, feels more like an object resting upon the chest. But it's definitely cooler than silicone, which heats up body temperature in a couple of minutes on a warm day. In a downpour, however, silicone has the edge. Wearing a Perma-Form bra while taking her daughter on a very rainy college tour, Lillie soon found that "my breasts were down around my waist." At such times, a woman's gotta do what a woman's gotta do. Lillie wrung 'em out. "A man saw me," she remembers, "and fell down the steps."

HANDLE WITH CARE

A prosthetic device needs care and attention. It should be washed with soap and water (monthly in the winter, weekly—or more often—in the sweat-inducing summer if it resides in a mastectomy bra with a pocket, and perhaps daily if it adheres to tape on her chest). After a washing, the prosthesis should be put back in the cradle it comes with to dry. In fact, it should rest in its cradle every night. That way it will hold its shape and won't be as likely to crack on the bottom early in its life. If your wife travels and forgets the cradle (a job for husbands: Remind her to take it), she can make a nest of clothes.

You may want to volunteer for laundry duty, if you're good with your hands. Your wife will undoubtedly be grateful, and I'm sure you'll have some funny stories to tell. Al Shockney would lay out his wife Lillie's Perma-Form bras for their air drying after a tumble in the washer. They were still on the basement poker table when his buddies came by for a card game. That night, the boys got a new sense of what it means to be a breast man.

As the silicone used in a prosthesis ages, it grows oozy and sticky—two adjectives that no one wants to hear applied to a breast. Insurance should cover a replacement every 2 years. It will also probably cover the cost of three special prosthesis bras the first year (they have a pouch for the ersatz breast), then at least one bra a year after that. But, as Hoyt says, "nobody wears one bra a year." She sells the bras for $42; they can cost up to $80 or so.

One more thing you should know: A prosthesis does have a habit of shifting.

After her bilateral mastectomy, TV journalist Linda Ellerbee reinvented her chest with saline implants. As she embarked on chemotherapy, an infection struck and the doctor had to remove the implants. She was planning to go back for a reimplantation, but first there was the matter of a vacation with her longtime companion Rolfe Tessem: a Caribbean getaway to celebrate the end of treatment. Ellerbee purchased Velcro prosthetic devices that could stick to adhesive tape she put on her chest. She thought she cut quite a dashing figure.

"I was so proud," she recalls. Tessem was sitting on his beach chair reading the *Wall Street Journal*, and Ellerbee trotted into the ocean for a swim, not ever considering how salt water, adhesive tape, and Velcro might interact.

The sun and surf felt great. After her swim, Ellerbee emerged from the water feeling like Bo Derek in the movie *Ten*. Only she couldn't help but notice that the man she loved, hiding behind the *Journal*, was shaking very hard as he struggled to keep from laughing. He appeared to be turning purple from the struggle to maintain a sober demeanor. Linda cast her gaze downward and discovered why he was laughing. One of her breasts was stuck on her hip and the other had slipped down to her butt.

"So much for Bo Derek," she says with a hearty laugh.

Twelve years later, Ellerbee and Tessem still laugh about the prosthetic debacle. And she hasn't been inclined to sign on for further adventures in breast replacement. Her chest is flat, she wears loose-fitting tops, and that's just fine with both of them.

"The most important lesson that Rolfe and I learned," Ellerbee says, "is that we both came to understand that we did not judge my femininity or my sexuality in terms of body parts." Besides, she says with a chuckle, her hiking backpack fits her much better now than it did before—you know, back when she had breasts.

RECONSTRUCTION

That's the term for the surgical re-creation of the lost breast. At best, reconstruction can produce a replacement breast that looks remarkably real. (If you don't believe me, type in "breast reconstruction and before-and-after" on

Google and take a look at some of those pictures.) Yet plastic surgeon Anne Nickodem, M.D., who practices in Virginia and Maryland, cautions that "there is no such thing as perfection."

Nor will the rebuilt breast function in the same way as its predecessor. A woman in her 40s or younger may eventually gain some sensation in the new breast—allowing her to feel hot or cold or the touch of a hand. But sexual sensation never returns. Some patients don't quite grasp that fact. Lillie Shockney is not surprised: "It looks so natural . . . it looks like a breast, it feels like a breast. So why doesn't it have sensation like a breast?" During the mastectomy, the nerve supply to the breast is severed. That's a clear loss for women who get a thrill from a breast caress.

Every woman who plans to undergo a mastectomy should be offered the option of reconstruction, and then decide for herself. And she shouldn't be afraid that reconstruction will interfere with the ability to detect recurrent breast cancer. "If it did, we wouldn't do it," says Richard Restifo, M.D., attending surgeon in the department of plastic surgery at Yale-New Haven Hospital in Connecticut. In addition, about 1 in 20 lumpectomy patients may see a significant change in the shape of their breasts because of the amount of tissue that is removed. They, too, might want to consider reconstructive surgery.

But in some parts of the country, plastic surgeons say, patients aren't routinely informed about reconstruction options. If your wife's surgeon is not able to refer you to a plastic surgeon who works with breast cancer patients, she might contact the American Society of Plastic Surgeons (www.plasticsurgery.org) for referrals.

At the initial meeting with a plastic surgeon, your wife will hear about the two basic procedures to consider: an implant, or a breast made of tissue taken from another part of her body. In the complicated world of breast cancer, wouldn't you know that Procedure A and Procedure B each has a couple of subsets, and all of the variations have their pros and cons. Your wife should understand what she's getting into. In almost every instance, several surgeries may be required before the new breast is deemed done. In addition, many women need surgery on the other breast—reduction or enhancement—to create symmetry. By law, health insurance has covered opposite breast surgery since 1999—both for patients who have reconstruction and for those who've had a large lumpectomy in one breast and need to have the other one reduced to match. It's a good idea to have a sample of the tissue removed from the other breast evaluated for "any unexpected cancer cells," suggests breast radiation oncologist Marisa Weiss, M.D., who practices in Philadelphia.

Your wife will also have to make a decision about the timing of the surgery. If the nature of her cancer gives her a high risk of recurrence, that may argue for delaying reconstruction until after chemotherapy and radiation. "For patients with stage III or IV breast cancer, most surgeons would prefer to delay the reconstruction by about a year," says Maurice Nahabedian, M.D., director of the plastic surgery group at the Johns Hopkins Breast Center in Baltimore. The goal is to complete treatments like chemotherapy and radiation and have a disease-free interval before beginning reconstruction.

Early-stage patients, however, can opt for "immediate reconstruction"—that is, right after the mastectomy. The advantage is an instant replacement for the lost breast. Some doctors believe that women don't suffer as much trauma over the mastectomy when the replacement is done without delay. The patient has one anesthetic experience and one hospitalization instead of two. Because scar tissue can develop if the woman has had radiation prior to reconstruction, sometimes it's harder for the plastic surgeon to obtain good results with an implant at a later date. But the decision is up to the doctor and your wife. "There's no 'right way,'" stresses Dr. Weiss. Your wife should quiz her team of docs to help her reach a decision that she's comfortable with. And no doctor should pressure your wife. Some newly diagnosed breast cancer patients feel that the last thing they want to face is a series of additional surgeries.

THE IMPLANT

Of the two types of reconstruction, the less complicated is the implant. The doctor can insert a saline or silicone breast implant under the pectoralis major muscle or first insert a "tissue expander," which does just what its name describes. The rubber balloonlike expander is pumped full of saline to stretch the skin on a weekly or every-other-week schedule. After 6 months or so, the patient is ready for the permanent implant.

GUY TALK

"Reconstructive surgery? She and I both felt that it wasn't that important. We feel the sense of one's beauty and of human emotions all come from within, not from without."

—WEI CHIN*, 45
whose wife, Betsy, had a mastectomy

Why opt for the expander? Surgeons like to remove as much breast tissue as possible, and then the skin needs to be stretched. Also, you know how when a surgically enhanced beach bunny lies down, her breasts don't lie down with her? That's what would happen if a larger-size implant were used without an expander. The expander creates a bigger pocket within which the implant can float. (Small-breasted women, however, may not need to go through the expander process and may be satisfied with a straightforward implant.)

As for the content of the permanent implant, your wife has a choice. Silicone gets everybody's vote as feeling more natural (and less sloshy) than saline. But silicone has a controversial history: Some patients have charged that silicone implant leakage has triggered autoimmune diseases. For the past few years, silicone implants have been available to breast cancer patients undergoing reconstruction if their plastic surgeon is participating in a clinical study. Your wife should discuss the matter with her surgeon.

She should also ask about the life span of an implant. No matter which she chooses—silicone or saline—any implant will eventually have to be replaced, usually in an outpatient procedure. The life span of an implant is 10 to 15 years, surgeons say. Either type of implant can rupture earlier. Saline leaks are easy to detect—the implant deflates. Silicone may leak from its capsule but stay in the breast area, making it more difficult to tell if there's been a rupture. Your wife should also think about the advantages of an implant. Women with young children might favor the implant because the recuperative period is shorter than for the tissue procedures. A dedicated athlete might also prefer the implant, which won't compromise abdominal or back strength like procedures that draw tissue from those parts of the body. The initial surgery takes about an hour, and the recovery time is about 3 weeks.

An implant, however, may not work for your wife. The maximum size is "large," which might still be too small to provide a matched set for some well-endowed women.

TAKING TISSUE

The other reconstruction option is to take tissue from another part of the body—the abdomen, back, or buttocks. Typically, the tissue is "tunneled" into its new position on the chest, but remains connected to its original blood vessels—that's "flap" reconstruction. In "free" reconstruction, the tissue is detached from blood vessels in its original site, then reattached to the blood vessels in the chest. The latter option, reserved for abdominal tissue, is a more difficult surgery but takes less of a toll on the stomach muscles.

Tissue reconstruction offers clear advantages over implants: a more natural-looking "breast," fashioned with a droop or slope to it; no worries about implants leaking or having to be replaced (although in some circumstances, particularly for the back procedure, an implant may have to be combined with surgery to give the new breast the appropriate volume). But the tissue procedure involves more complex surgery—90 minutes to 2 hours for the back tissue, 4 or 5 hours for abdominal tissue. Your wife will have two wounds that need to heal. In addition, complications can arise: abdominal weakness if the abdominal muscle is used, fat necrosis (the death of tissue, which needs to be repaired in additional surgery), and others.

Among plastic surgeons, abdominal tissue is currently the number one choice. Women tend to have enough tissue for a successful reconstruction, the tissue feels similar to breast tissue, and there's the added benefit of a tummy tuck.

There are three abdominal options: conventional TRAM flap, free TRAM flap, and DIEP flap. The most commonly performed is the conventional TRAM flap (the "t" stands for "transverse," a reference to the incision and scar that stretches from hip to hip; the "ram" stands for the *rectus abdominus* muscle that is moved in the surgery). The free TRAM takes a smaller portion of the abdominal muscle. The newer DIEP flap reconstruction uses no muscle at all but is a more difficult surgery to perform. The doctor severs the abdominal tissues but aims to spare the muscle, then reconnects the tissue via microsurgery. DIEP, by the way, stands for "deep inferior epigastric perforator," which is really more than you need to know. But you do need to know that a plastic surgeon should have ample experience with this procedure. Your wife may have to travel to one of the relatively small number of centers that do the DIEP. To find a list of doctors who perform this type of reconstruction, check the Web site www.carlopress.com/141/cat141.htm?14. If she has the surgery out of town, she should expect to stay put for 7 to 10 days, or until all of the drains are removed.

Doctors can get good results from all three kinds of abdominal operations, although abdominal strength is significantly compromised with the conventional TRAM procedure. The removal of the abdominal muscles can also cause an abdominal bulge or hernia in a small percentage of patients (the insertion of a piece of mesh during the procedure can reduce the chances of such complications). On the pain index, the conventional TRAM flap ranks highest and the DIEP lowest because there is minimal violation of muscles. In all cases, patients typically walk hunched over for about a week.

Moving muscle from the back—the *latissimus dorsi*—has taken, um, a back seat to the popular abdominal procedures. The back tissue and muscle is not quite the same texture as a breast, and, as I mentioned, a patient who has little fat on her back may need an implant to gain the appropriate volume to match the other breast. But the complication rate is reportedly lower for this procedure.

The buttocks are favored as a tissue source in certain centers. A woman who'd like to shed a few pounds in her posterior might find this procedure appealing. But breastcancer.org, in its very helpful rundown of the various reconstruction options, notes that "buttocks crease transfer surgery is rarely done because of its complexity and high failure rate."

THE CHOICE IS HERS

As I interviewed plastic surgeons, I came to see that each had his or her favorite among the reconstruction procedures. "That is absolutely true," says Dr. Nahabedian. Your wife should be aware of a doctor's biases. Researching the options beforehand might help her decide which surgery is most suitable for her. (The Web site www.breastcancer.org has thorough assessments of each method of reconstruction.)

Most husbands take the proper breast cancer husband stand: Whatever you want, dear. When the husband dominates the conversation, says Dr. Nahabedian, "that worries me. I try to figure out whom she's doing it for."

If you find yourself pushing your wife toward reconstruction, consider this: What if she goes ahead with the surgery and there are complications, and you're the one who wanted it?

"The best role for the husband is to be there if his wife needs him to interpret things, to ask questions," says Dr. Olding. "At the end of the appointment, if he has questions, he should ask them, but it's the wife who has to make the decisions."

That's why the doctor should be locking eyes with your wife, and not you. Indeed, the surgeon's personality may play a part in her decision. Jim Finkelstein and his wife, Laurie Ferreri, visited four plastic surgeons to discuss reconstruction. The first three doctors talked to Jim directly instead of addressing Laurie. One doc even got into a conversation with Jim about golf. The fourth doctor talked to Laurie and just about ignored Jim. That's the surgeon they selected—and, of course, that's the way all of your cancer doctors should talk to both of you.

With additional surgery, the doctor can "reconstruct" (via tissue and/or tattoo) the nipple and areola. Some women are fine without these finishing touches, or opt for less permanent fixtures like paste-on nipples. Others are raring to go. "I'm going for broke, and I want it all," laughs Lillie Shockney, 50, who had her reconstruction years after her mastectomies. "When am I getting my nip, nip, nipples?" she teases her plastic surgeon, sounding for all the world like a kid eagerly awaiting a Christmas Barbie.

Of course, there's more to it than that. For many women, reconstruction is a way of reclaiming what was lost to breast cancer. "It goes back to what your relationship is with your breast," says Shockney.

Before your wife makes any decision, she might want to look at the doctor's book of befores and afters. If the afters are all gorgeous, then your wife is not getting a realistic view of the range of outcomes. She should see a range of body types, from petite to portly. Keep in mind that before-and-after books usually won't show what happens, say, 5 years down the road. As the natural breast droops, its reconstructed partner will stay, for lack of a better word, perky.

RECUPERATION

When Dr. Nickodem emerges from a reconstruction surgery, she heads to the waiting room to tell the husband how things went and how long his wife will have to stay in the hospital. Then she'll ask, "Any questions?"

"The big question from husbands is, 'How soon can we have sex?'" she reports. She feels like telling them, "Do you get the big picture? Your wife has breast cancer. She just lost her breast. She underwent a 5½-hour surgery, and you want to know *when she can have sex?"*

THE POST-RECONSTRUCTION WORKOUT

Your wife may be focusing on the cosmetics of her surgery, and that's perfectly understandable. But you should encourage her to ask the plastic surgeon about the surgery's impact on her quality of life. When reconstructive surgery uses abdominal or back muscle to build a new breast, her body will not work the same way. Abdominal muscles support the back. Back muscles play a role in actions such as getting up from a seated position. Performing certain exercises can prevent problems after these surgeries. "I feel it is very important to ask, 'If you take the muscle, is there something I should do to compensate?'" suggests physical therapist Janet Sobel, who practices in the Washington, D.C., area and works with many breast cancer patients.

Your wife won't need to make a huge commitment of time—physical therapy and home exercises for 6 weeks, then a maintenance program. But without the proper postsurgery exercises, Sobel believes, a woman may experience unnecessary pain and weakness later on. To get a good idea of what to expect, your wife also might ask the surgeon if she can speak with a patient who has gone through the same surgery. That way she can hear a firsthand account of life after reconstruction.

Dr. Nickodem sometimes teases her patients, "If you need a 6-month prescription for no sex, let me know."

So, maybe that's a question you shouldn't ask your wife's plastic surgeon, at least not right away. But in case you're wondering, you and your wife can typically resume relations 3 to 4 weeks after an implant or a back flap procedure, and more like 6 weeks after an abdominal procedure. That is, *if she feels up to it.*

Here's what else you need to know: For at least 3 weeks following an implant or back procedure, and for 6 to 8 weeks after a TRAM flap, your wife will be recuperating. She will not go back to work. She will be prohibited from lifting while healing. You will be the chief cook and dishwasher (and laundry man and more). If friends and family are offering a hand, now's the time to accept—or to hire help if you have the budget.

Your wife will also need you in other ways. "The norm is to step up to the plate, to change the dressings, to empty bloody drainage bulbs," says Dr. Nickodem. "Many husbands say, 'I don't think I can do this.' You'll be surprised what you'll be able to do." If your wife is reluctant to expose her scars to you, she suggests that you might say, "I don't mind, honey, let me help you. We'll get through this together." That is, unless you're the kind of guy who faints at the sight of a scar.

And, of course, a nice gift never hurts. Dr. Nickodem has seen husbands surprise their wives with trips to Italy or a gift certificate to a spa. "It doesn't have to be something big," she adds. "Just doing something very simple for your wife makes a world of difference."

THE AFTERMATH

Post-surgery, you may think your wife's breast looks fine, and she may not. Family members might tell her, "You have two breasts—what's the problem?" Yet she may feel that, well, it's not the same. It's possible she'll obsess about the scarring if she had a flap procedure; or she'll be unhappy that her belly button is off center if she had a procedure that drew fat from her abdomen. Be patient, counsels Shockney. Your wife may need to go through a yearlong cycle, all the holidays and seasons, to get to the point where she feels comfortable with her new breast.

If all goes well, your wife will be one of the majority: women who are happy with their reconstruction. But not every woman is pleased with the outcome. "I don't know if I would do it again," says Alice Todd*, who opted for a tissue expander followed by an implant after her mastectomy 6 years ago. "I didn't realize how much surgery was involved; they don't tell you everything." (Or maybe they did, and the Todds were suffering from the common affliction of breast cancer information overload.)

Her husband, Harry, encouraged her to have the surgery, thinking she'd "feel better about herself, her clothing, and everything else."

He pauses. "To be honest, I don't think she's very happy with the way it went."

"I'm not at all," Alice admits.

"It just didn't turn out that great," Harry explains. After 6 years, the reconstructed left breast is tight and firm, and the right breast is "lower and bigger."

Alice never bothered to have her nipple reconstructed. "It was enough surgery. I was tired of being a pin cushion." Besides, she says, Harry is the only one who knows. And he doesn't mind.

READY OR NOT?

There's no statute of limitations on reconstruction. Dr. Nahabedian of Johns Hopkins told me of a 68-year-old breast cancer survivor who came by 25 years after her first mastectomy. She had just had a breast cancer diagnosis in the other breast, and she wanted that side to be reconstructed. He asked her, "What about the other side?"

"I didn't think you could do anything," she said. "No one ever told me."

To her surprise, it wasn't too late to have a matching set.

Some women who initially don't want reconstruction get fed up with the hassle of a prosthesis. Lillie Shockney waited over 10 years for reconstruction; her problems tolerating anesthesia had prevented the surgery earlier. After so long, her husband didn't quite understand why she felt the need to have the reconstructive surgery. Did he do something wrong?

It was so unlike her, she admits, to do something for herself and herself alone. "I told him that he has been wonderful, but that I missed my breasts," Shockney says. "I missed my cleavage. I didn't feel comfortable being on top facing him and not feeling the pendulum swing of my breasts. I wanted to wear whatever clothes I wished to without limitations. I then asked him to tell me the truth as to whether he missed them, too. He bowed his head and said, 'Yes,' without eye contact. That made me cry, but they were happy tears."

Jim Zabora, Sc.D., dean of the School of Social Service at the Catholic University of America in Washington, D.C., tells a poignant story that shows how the issues that surround a mastectomy—and the possibility of reconstruction—may linger for years.

A group of Baltimore men would take their wives to a breast cancer support group at a local community college. Men being men, they'd sit silently in the lobby, reading the sports page or twiddling their thumbs while their wives poured out their hearts in a classroom down the hall. Zabora figured he had the perfect setup to start a men's support group. While the wives had their session, he led the husbands in theirs. Since the wives had seen a film about reconstruction and talked about it, Zabora decided to show the same movie to the husbands. When it was over, one man—a fire chief—broke down sobbing.

Zabora offered to take him aside and talk, but the man wanted to let everyone in the group know what was troubling him. (See, sometimes guys do want to talk about their feelings.) His wife did not have reconstruction after her mastectomy 2 years ago, he explained to his fellow breast cancer husbands. He had always told her that it didn't matter to him. That he loved her and not her breasts. But watching the movie, he realized that he missed the missing breast. He did want her to have reconstruction. And he didn't know how to tell her all this, because he had always said that it didn't matter.

Whew.

"The biggest thing was to open up communication," Zabora says. "The men in the group worked with him to figure out what he could say when he got home." They suggested he wait for his wife to bring up the video on reconstruction. And then ask, "What do you think about that video? Is that something you've thought about?"

Zabora knows that the fire chief broached the subject, but he doesn't know how the story ends.

I was intrigued by this story. So were psychologists and social workers with whom I shared the account.

"It's good to be able to talk about it," says psychologist Beth Meyerowitz, Ph.D., a professor of psychology and preventive medicine at the University of Southern California in Los Angeles. "But there's a big difference between saying, 'You really ought to have reconstruction,' and 'I've been thinking about something—have you?'"

But should the fire chief have raised the subject at all? I wondered if he would be putting his wife in a very difficult position, because once he says he'd like her to think about reconstruction, wouldn't she be feeling a little pressured? "It's very difficult," says Roz Kleban, a social worker at Memorial Sloan-Kettering in New York City, who runs support groups for breast cancer patients. "I would work with him to see if he can cope with the fact that the breast is missing. And I would want him to work on accepting things as they are. Because she should not do it for him. She should only do it for herself."

BOOB JOKES

Despite the agony of facing a mastectomy, and the overwhelming array of options for replacing the lost breast, husbands and wives do find humor in the matter.

One fellow nicknamed his wife's reconstructed breast "Frankenboob." Even a prosthesis can get a name—Lillie Shockney dubbed hers "Betty Boob."

David Freeman remembers how he laughed at the very idea of a reconstruction that drew fat from the abdomen. The doctor told his wife that she'd have perky young breasts and a free tummy tuck, too. "Hey, this is all good," Freeman thought.

And then there's the guy who told me how his wife playfully sizes up her two breasts, the recently reconstructed one and the real one. "25, 40; 25, 40," she'll laugh, assigning an age to the youthful-looking fake and to its less-youthful real partner.

What can you say but . . . surreal.

TIPS ➢ ➢ ➢

1. Different plastic surgeons have different preferences when it comes to reconstruction: implants, back tissue, abdominal tissue, butt tissue. Your wife should research the options so she can form her own opinion rather than be swayed by a doctor's bias.
2. There's no time limit on when reconstruction can be done. If your wife is not interested at present, you (and her doctors) should respect her opinion.
3. Be prepared to pitch in at home if your wife has reconstructive surgery. It will take several weeks for her to recuperate.

➢ BONUS TIP

The plastic surgeon may suggest reducing or enlarging your wife's unaffected breast for a better match with its reconstructed partner. The resultant scarring and calcifications could mimic early cancer, creating mammogram angst in the future that needs to be resolved with a biopsy. This isn't a reason to forego opposite breast surgery, but it is a good reason for a baseline mammogram 6 months after reconstruction.

The Intimate Details

Everything you always wanted to know about sex and breast cancer

"We had oral sex," says David Moyer about the months when his wife, Brenda, was feeling worn down by chemo and not at all in the mood for love. "We just talked about it."

Well, at least they were talking.

There are two big taboos in conversations about breast cancer. One is death. The other is sex.

Why the silence?

Your wife's doctors are busy saving her life with surgery and chemotherapy and radiation. They may feel they don't have time to raise the subject of a patient's sex life. Or they might be a little uncomfortable asking. At a breast cancer forum in Philadelphia, a social worker asked a room packed with dozens of women (and a few devoted husbands) if their cancer docs had ever mentioned sex to them. By my count, three people raised their hands.

Breast cancer patients may not be inclined to put sex at the top of their "must-discuss" list, either. They're afraid for their lives, and they're coping with the ill effects of the treatments they must endure. And if they've lost a breast or their hair, you can bet they're not feeling especially sexy.

And then there are the husbands. Yup, there we are. We've still got our 9-to-whenever jobs. Except now we may be taking time off to run to doctor's appointments with our wives. And we're probably picking up some of the household slack—driving carpools, shopping for groceries, folding laundry, and the like. So we're pretty busy. Not to mention frightened, too. Yet we've still got our sex drive. Here's how Vern Taylor, 52, of Winnipeg sums up his sexual feelings after his wife, Susan, 51, was diagnosed with breast cancer 6 years ago: "You are still exactly the same man you were. Your hormones haven't changed. If you wanted sex 10 times last week, you still want it. My testosterone was saying, 'You better have sex.' But, oops, I'm married. It better be with my wife. Oh, she's not interested. You have to kind of park it."

That's why many breast cancer husbands are even afraid to flirt. They don't want their poor wives to think they're pressuring them to have sex, so they pull back. Which makes their wives think they're not sexy anymore.

Talk about a lose–lose situation.

SEX BEFORE AND AFTER SURGERY

My wife and I were among the lucky ones. After her oncologist told us all the terrible things that chemotherapy can do to a body—namely, that it would transform my wife into a bald, queasy, pale ghost of herself—he said in a low, gentle voice, "but you can maintain intimacy during this period."

To which I wanted to say, "Doc, you've got to be kidding!"

He wasn't. In retrospect, Marsha and I are deeply thankful that he planted the thought in our heads that cancer and chastity aren't synonymous.

But just as treatments for breast cancer have many variations, a couple's sexual relations will play out in different ways.

For many couples, the period immediately after diagnosis is a time when sex is not on anyone's mind. You and your wife are no doubt in shock, running from doctor to doctor, processing information about the tumor, figuring out what to do. Needless to say, none of these activities are conducive to romance. Still, sex doesn't fall into a black hole forever. As your wife makes decisions about treatment, some of the stress diminishes. You or she may be feeling a little frisky. There may even be a bit of dark humor involved as you do it. Lili Romero-DeSimone remembers "farewell to my boob sex" before her mastectomy.

Following surgery, making whoopee is usually not at the top of the to-do list. If your wife has had a mastectomy or a dissection of the nodes under her armpit, she will come home with a drainage bulb or two dangling from the incision. I was fairly certain that no woman would want to fool around while trailing a bulb. But never underestimate the power of sexual desire. "Oh yes, I've known people who had sex then," says Kyle Terrell, a surgical oncology nurse practitioner at the Johns Hopkins Breast Center in Baltimore. The woman might want to be on the bottom, Terrell demurely advises, so, um, you know, her drainage bulbs don't swing around during intercourse.

(I think this is a good moment to pass on an important "pubic service" message from my wife: If your beloved is not interested in sex when she's dangling bulbs, or recuperating from surgery, or suffering through chemo, why, then, too bad for you.)

After a couple of weeks, the drainage bulbs will be gone. Perhaps your wife won't need chemo or hasn't yet begun that stage of treatment. If you're both in the mood, there's no reason not to have sex. Scars can even serve as an aphrodisiac, at least for some men. On the Web site www.breastcancer.org, one fellow posted a note: "I want to move my tongue along the thin white line of her incision."

More typically, men are nervous about recommencing sex after surgery. They're afraid. Can I touch this? Can I do that? Will I hurt my wife?

"There's a real possibility for a downward spiral," says Beth Meyerowitz, Ph.D., a professor of psychology and preventive medicine at the University of Southern California who does research on cancer survivors and their partners. The husband may be thinking, "I'm not going to focus on the breast. I don't want to hurt her. I don't want to make her feel it's the most important thing."

The wife, meanwhile, may be thinking, "He's not touching my chest the way he used to. He must be disgusted." So she pulls away. And he thinks he made overtures too soon. Attempting to be thoughtful, he may say, "We don't need to do this."

"I say to women, men aren't mind readers," says Mary Jane Massie,

GUY TALK

"The kind of sex that figures in right after something like cancer is a quieter kind of sex. Maybe you're not bouncing off the walls. But it turns out to be the best kind of sex."

—MICHAEL TUCKER, 60
Mill Valley, California

M.D., a psychiatrist who sees patients at Memorial Sloan-Kettering Cancer Center in New York City. "If the man is avoiding sex, it is often because he is frightened. Take your husband's hand and put it on your chest. Tell him, 'If you touch here and here, it doesn't hurt. But here it's a little tender.'"

Guys, if you're afraid to touch, tell your wives what Dr. Massie said.

After her surgery (and minus any drainage bulbs), your wife may prefer to be on top during sex. That lets her set the agenda, explains Megan Mills, Ph.D., director of psychosocial oncology at Chicago's Rush Cancer Institute. On top, she can decide how active to be, how far to go. She is in control. The husband also benefits from the arrangement. "He doesn't have to worry about when it's too much," Dr. Mills says. "The wife is in a position to let you know."

For aquatic-minded couples with a backyard pool, Dr. Mills proposes swimming pool sex. "Making love in water is much easier on everybody," she says. "I think it has to do with buoyancy. Women who've had breast surgery might be worried about supporting themselves with their arms. They might be afraid of setting off lymphedema—the arm swelling that can occur after the removal of lymph nodes. Those fears may vanish in a pool."

Dr. Mills pauses and laughs. "You should have seen the faces on this Baptist minister and his wife when I said that."

And if your wife has had a mastectomy and is feeling self-conscious? "I felt so terrible when I lost my breasts," remembers Cookie Medansky of Chicago, a 19-year breast cancer survivor who was diagnosed at age 47 and had a double mastectomy. Her husband, Earl, put her at ease. "He told me the most important part was there, and he'd find something else to do with his hands." He also bought her pretty silk camisoles so she'd feel better about getting intimate.

That's exactly what the experts recommend for a couple when the woman has had a mastectomy and is feeling a little tentative about unveiling herself. "First, you buy her a peignoir—really sexy, short lingerie," Dr. Mills says. And the room should be romantically lit, almost dark. That takes the focus off the breast.

SHIFTING THE FOCUS

If you really want to take the focus off the breast, Dr. Mills suggests the classic Masters and Johnson sex therapy technique called "sensate focus." The idea is to set aside a series of evenings to learn about what turns each other on, but without any pressure to perform.

Not every husband and wife would be comfortable with sensate focus. But if you're intrigued, I'll give you a condensed course.

For the first session, you and your wife doff your clothes. Each of you will take turns being the toucher and the touchee. Be a gentleman and let your wife go first. You lie back on the bed. Your wife can caress your body with her fingers, kiss with her lips, tickle with a feather. But no contact with breasts or genitals. You have to tell your wife what you find sensuous and what you find uncomfortable—and what tickles. Don't be cranky and whine, "You do this all the time and I really hate it," Dr. Mills suggests. Be constructive and specific: "It would feel better if you applied more pressure or less pressure." After 30 minutes, switch roles.

In the second session, you can touch the breast and genitals, but only briefly and lightly—and still no touching to the point of orgasm. "Guiding a partner's hand is especially helpful with genital caressing, because it is often difficult to explain your desires in words," notes sex therapist Leslie Schover, Ph.D., whose enlightening book *Sexuality and Fertility After Cancer* discusses sensate focus, among many other things.

Then comes the third session, during which "you can ask the giver to prolong the sexual touching until you have an orgasm," according to Dr. Schover.

Or not.

The idea is not to rush into anything, to learn to talk about sex instead of focusing on orgasm, and to understand what each of you finds erotic.

That's what actor Michael Tucker came to understand after his wife was diagnosed with breast cancer in 1986. At the time, Tucker and his wife, Jill Eikenberry, were starring in the hit show *L.A. Law*. Tucker's TV character, Stuart Markowitz, was renowned for a sexual technique called the Venus Butterfly that guaranteed an amazing degree of satisfaction. The Butterfly was a figment of an *L.A. Law* writer's overheated imagination. After his wife's surgery and radiation, Tucker invented a real-life Butterfly—a new way to practice the joy of sex.

"The best sex for a man is to please his woman," says Tucker. "Now that sounds like an obvious statement, but after years of chasing my own pleasure and coming up a little bit short, I realized that if I could give her everything she ever wanted and more, I felt like a million bucks." That's everything *she* wants and not what you think she wants. How do you know? You ask. "We do talk a lot about sex," Tucker says. And both partners benefit. Instead of "obligatory sex," he says, the husband gets to a stage where he'll never have to ask, "What about me?" again.

"It turns out," Tucker says, "to be the best kind of sex."

CHEMO AND COUPLING

Fortunately, the Tuckerberries, as they call themselves, didn't have to face the rigors of chemo. Because chemotherapy and sex are definitely not a match made in heaven. "Most sexual activity decreases during chemotherapy because people are fatigued," says Patricia Ganz, M.D., an oncologist who is professor of health services and medicine at the UCLA Schools of Medicine and Public Health. Plus, for the first 24 hours after an infusion, having intercourse or oral sex with your wife might not be advisable. The chemotherapy drugs may be secreted through the vaginal mucosa and could cause a rash on the penis (although probably not any long-term problems). Even in the closest of marriages, the husband doesn't need to share his wife's dose. The solution is simply to wait a day or so. Or if neither of you feels like waiting, a condom should offer protection.

Beyond these physical barriers to sex, there are emotional ones as well. "For a young woman who has just found out that her chemo may make her infertile, thinking about having sex is more likely to make her cry than to turn her on," says Dr. Schover, who is a professor of behavioral science in the cancer prevention division at the University of Texas M.D. Anderson Cancer Center in Houston.

In addition, chemotherapy can cause mucositis—an inflammation of the mucous membranes lining the mouth and the vagina. In such cases, sexual intercourse can be painful.

Yet sex may still be possible—and comfortable—for many women going through chemo. Your wife may have relatively mild side effects, and, as Bethesda, Maryland, psychologist Venus Masselam, Ph.D., puts it, "If there's a way that sex can happen, and it's not painful, and it doesn't feel abusive to either person, it's an important thing to maintain."

"Your wife may have a couple of good days in that chemo period," says Edwin Cotto, 43, of Garfield, New Jersey, whose wife was diagnosed with breast cancer twice, first in the left breast, then in the right breast 5 years later. "Then, like when you're dating, you try to see if you can get some. If it didn't happen, it didn't happen. I'm not going to die."

But instead of asking, many men pull back.

In support groups, Jean Lynn, an oncology nurse who is program director for the Breast Care Center at George Washington University Medical Faculty Associates in Washington, D.C., has heard men say, "I just thought she wasn't interested."

Lynn asks them, "How would you feel if you lost all your hair and had a disfiguring scar? Would you feel sexually desirable?" And wouldn't you want your wife to let you know you still were the apple of her eye?

That raises the inevitable question: How do you come on to a woman when she's undergoing chemo?

Gently, without sending any signals that she'll let you down if she's not up to it. You might have your own manly perspective ("Me want sex"), but she might crave nothing more than a good cuddle.

On a day when your wife is feeling okay, put your arm around her and head to the bedroom. If your wife's parents or siblings are staying with you, treat them to movie tickets. (Otherwise, you might end up like one couple who was beset with houseguests during the wife's cancer siege; they "fooled around" in the bedroom closet.) If you've got kids and they're at home, farm them out—people want to help, so let them.

And then . . . Well, I can tell you how it happened for Marsha and me. My wife felt exquisitely self-conscious about the whole thing, what with being bald and all. Marsha was so embarrassed by her hairless state that she wanted to at least keep her wig on while we made love. I told her, "No, it's me." So she removed her crown of hair. With her lovely egg-shaped head, she had an exotic beauty, like an exquisite space alien. And so we did it, with a tip o' the hat to Astroglide, an over-the-counter lubricant that can remedy the vaginal dryness caused by chemo. (One sexually active couple in their 70s told nurse Jean Lynn that "Crisco works as well and is a lot cheaper." The experts I interviewed had one word: "Yuck.")

As the months of chemo wore on, Marsha felt less and less like having sex—a common phenomenon. "Life changes during chemotherapy for everyone, for the partner as well as the patient," says Dr. Ganz. "Acknowledge that this is when you will have downtime in terms of a lot of activities that were normal. But that your wife will get better and you will resume those activities."

AN "OWNER-OPERATOR"

The breast cancer husbands I interviewed were okay with temporary abstinence. "I have this funny feeling that if I felt the need, Carol would say 'yes' because that's the way she is. But I felt like it would have been an imposition on her. Her body was all screwed up from chemo," says Phil Gay, 63, a strapping retired navy captain who now works as a fly-fishing guide. "And I'm used to going on deployment for 8 or 9 months. Being abstinent is not a big deal for me."

"Basically, you have to make that part of your life private," Vern Taylor reflects. "It's your responsibility if you want to run it, and don't feel bad. You are a healthy man."

That is to say: Yes, breast cancer husbands do masturbate. In the words of a truck driver whose wife found sex too painful to think about: "Sometimes, you have to be an owner-operator."

Obviously, this is a personal choice. "I think masturbation is perfectly normal," says Dr. Schover. "In couples where the desire for sex isn't exactly equal, it's a great way to make sure each person is satisfied without putting a lot of stress on the other."

You can tell your wife. Or you can keep quiet.

But even if you are, ahem, running your own sex life while your wife suffers through chemo, she still craves an intimate touch. "The loss of touch is just the biggest loss we can experience," says Dr. Masselam. "There's nothing like a foot rub with a nice cream. There are so many other ways of connecting that we totally omit. The repertoire is so limited."

RECONNECTING

If you stop touching altogether, you could face a much harder time when you and your wife are ready to reconnect. Sure, that first encounter after a long hiatus might be wonderful—like falling in love all over again. Or it might be as awkward as a teenager's first kiss.

I met a charming woman in her early 30s who was just finishing up her treatment. She was ready for action, but her husband told her the months of inactivity had put his libido on ice.

"Sounds fishy to me," says Dr. Schover. "He probably has a lot of anxieties. And it's nice and easy to blame her—'because of your illness and because we didn't have sex, you wrecked me as a man.'" Or perhaps the husband was afraid of hurting his wife.

In what I would deem an ironic twist, the same young woman whose husband had lost his sex drive told me that a vacation from canoodling wouldn't be a problem for older couples who've gone through breast cancer. She figured that for the AARP generation, sex is just a memory.

She and her husband could take a lesson from 67-year-old Dick Greenberg and his 56-year-old wife, Carla.

Carla's sexual desire had just started returning following chemotherapy; Dick made inquiries. Carla wasn't feeling quite ready, but "the sexual act was never repugnant," she says. And she liked the fact that Dick had propositioned her. "He always just said, 'You are beautiful.' He never flinched looking at the lumpectomy scar. He still desired me even though chemo doesn't make you the sexiest woman on the street. So I always felt I was desirable, and that helps a lot—even if you're not getting what I call 'the big O.'" Besides, she liked the cuddling and hugging.

As Dr. Schover puts it, "I think it's perfectly fine for couples to sometimes have a sexual encounter where one person reaches orgasm and the other doesn't."

Other women want to take it slowly—very slowly—and that might lead to tensions. When I met Sally Estefan* and her husband, Rick, she had endured a mastectomy and months of chemotherapy, and was in the middle of

---

TOY STORY

At conferences on breast cancer, Philadelphia breast radiation oncologist Marisa Weiss, M.D., encourages women who've gone through treatment to visit a sex-toy store in search of new play-things to perk up their sexual relationship with hubbie.

"There are all kinds of outfits and things that speak to fantasy," she says. "One thing that can help you go from here (that is, no sex) to there (back in the saddle again) is the power of your mind. And fantasy is important. There's a whole area of erotica that you never even considered before that might help you get in the mood."

Dr. Weiss has a suitcase full of tricks that she brings to her "Sex After Breast Cancer: Tips and Toys" workshop. To find toys that you and your wife enjoy, Dr. Weiss suggests taking a trip to a sex novelty shop or heading to the Internet. One breast cancer survivor, for example, now wears "Buzz Me Panties" from the Toys in Babeland catalog or www.babeland.com. When her husband is in the mood, he uses the remote control that comes with the panties to give her a buzz. (She lets him know if she's in the mood, too.)

Some creative turn-ons don't require toys. One of Dr. Weiss's breast cancer patients acts out her husband's fantasy. He goes to a bar first. She comes in later all gussied up, acting like a stranger. He picks her up; they go home and have hot sex.

radiation. Her hair was beginning to grow back—a nubby cap of blond fuzz. Her sexual desire was beginning to return as well.

During chemotherapy, Sally lived a celibate life. "Sexual intimacy has been nonexistent since I was diagnosed," she said. "I had the recovery from my mastectomy and then chemo. If I wasn't nauseated, chemo had eradicated my estrogen. Sex is excruciatingly painful."

So she didn't miss it.

"I just kinda put it on the back burner," Rick says. "I got fatter."

"And he also masturbates," Sally says matter-of-factly.

She'd like to have sex with him, but she says, "I feel totally not sexy. It's hard for me to feel sexy. And my feeling is, can I hold onto my man if I can't be sexual? I don't think a man can survive without sex."

"Don't ask me, man," Rick says. "I don't know. I've been revirginated."

But now, Sally says, she'd like to try, for lack of a better term, fooling around. Not sexual intercourse just yet. Maybe just making out. "But I'm afraid to ask because I don't want to have sex."

Actually, she did ask once. Rick passed. "I was tired," he says.

And he pauses. "The problem with guys is, you start it and you want to finish it."

A sex therapist would point out that if you don't at least start, you'll never get a chance to finish.

Besides, a husband could be facing a far bleaker outlook. Dr. Massie at Memorial Sloan-Kettering recalls how, to her horror, "A woman in her 50s said to me, 'The one good thing about breast cancer is I will never have to do that again. I've got the trump excuse!'"

WHEN LOVE HURTS

As was the case with Sally, many women who go through chemotherapy experience vaginal dryness and find sex painful—even after treatment is over. In addition, their sex drive may be diminished, which is what happens when women are pushed into menopause by chemotherapy.

Women who take tamoxifen, the estrogen-blocking pill, often lay the blame on the medication. But that may not be the real reason. In a study comparing postmenopausal breast cancer survivors with a similar group of postmenopausal women without breast cancer, complaints about vaginal dryness were "exactly the same" in each group, says Dr. Ganz. "The pain associated with sex is probably from menopause-related vaginal dryness. But they're attributing it to tamoxifen." (Yet she is careful to note that tamoxifen can cause subtle sexual problems, though vaginal discharge is more common than vaginal dryness.)

Then there's the group of already-menopausal women who, upon diagnosis, stopped hormone replacement therapy. Stopping HRT can cause vaginal dryness. For these physical reasons, as well as psychological reasons, "sexual problems occur with considerable frequency in breast cancer patients," Dr. Ganz wrote in a recent paper, "and extend beyond the acute phase of treatment."

One over-the-counter solution is Replens, a vaginal moisturizer that the woman uses regularly, even if she's not having sex. There is also an array of water-based lubricants sold at drugstores as well as through Web sites like drugstore.com, evesgarden.com, and goodvibes.com. When you (or your wife) are shopping for lubricants, Dr. Schover points out that the newer, thinner liquids like K-Y Silk-E and Astroglide "feel much more natural and stay slippery longer without drying out and getting tacky like gels."

The need for a lubricant may put a crimp in spontaneity, but really, what's the alternative? "If you are only willing to do what was done in the past, it's going to pose problems," says Dorothy Davis, 53, of Bowie, Maryland, a breast cancer survivor. "You have to be open and willing to experiment."

Foreplay, for example, takes a little more time since Dorothy only has one breast with sexual sensation. (The other breast is a post-mastectomy reconstruction.) And even lubricants require some getting used to.

"In the winter time, that stuff is cold," says her husband John, 55.

"Not just in the winter time," Dorothy says. "It is co-o-o-o-old."

"Let me tell you what we did," she continues. "We got a baby bottle warmer and keep it by the bed, and keep our K-Y in the water."

"When the bottle warmer goes 'beep, beep,'" John says, "we're like Pavlov's dog." (Another option might be to try K-Y Warming Liquid Personal Lubricant, which warms upon bodily contact.)

If gels, jellies, and lubricants aren't enough to alleviate your wife's vaginal dryness, doctors do have other solutions. But first, someone has to bring up the topic. "I ask about vaginal dryness," says Dr. Ganz—a low-key way to broach the subject. If your doctor doesn't make the first move, your wife can raise the issue.

The remedies aren't perfect, and they're not appropriate for every patient. But you should at least discuss them. Vaginal estrogens can keep the vagina stretchy and lubricated, although it has no clear influence on sexual desire or pleasure. Testosterone—delivered orally or via patch—does little for the genitals but acts in the brain to promote desire for sex.

Testosterone is the more controversial therapy. "Some people in the field of sexuality treatment are just stuck on testosterone as the answer to everything," says Dr. Schover. But it is unclear how much testosterone women need for "normal desire"—or whether testosterone levels are related to level of sexual desire in postmenopausal women. In addition, some doctors worry that high testosterone levels are actually a risk factor for breast cancer.

Even though estrogen is seemingly the last thing you'd want to give a breast cancer survivor, since it fuels tumors classified as hormone receptor-positive, some doctors will sign off on estrogen delivered to the vagina. One delivery method is the Estring, a plastic ring inserted in the vagina that slowly dispenses estrogen. Vagifem tablets also emit a low level of estrogen. In addition, there are vaginal estrogen creams, although oncologists may not like them because the dose that gets into the bloodstream is less predictable than with Estring or Vagifem. "Creams can give a woman a whopping dose of estrogen," Dr. Schover says.

Yet for some couples, nothing seems to work. "Let me tell you, Heather has literally had no desire. Period," says Dan Fields*, 46. "I mean, it has stopped. When that tamoxifen kicked in, it was like she didn't want to be around as far as sexual intercourse. And the doctor told me she is so dry that I could tear her. That's all he needed to tell me."

"We're wrestling with the issue," says Heather, 42. "Chemo did not throw me into menopause, so Arimidex [a postmenopausal hormonal therapy] is not an option. The doctor said, 'You guys have to make a quality of life decision' about staying on tamoxifen." Doctors have told her that her extreme sensitivity to medications may be responsible; that's little solace.

Dan, meanwhile, has no doubts about his stance: "I'm never going to be the reason she is taken off tamoxifen."

But many couples are able to resume their sex lives. In fact, some even expand their repertoire as a result of breast cancer treatment. Lillie Shockney, the forthright Johns Hopkins nurse, tells of a couple she counseled. The wife was having a mastectomy and reconstruction that would take tissue from the abdomen. Shockney gave them the ground rules: oral sex permissible after 3 weeks (when the stomach and breast are still healing), vaginal sex after 6. The wife dutifully wrote everything down.

After the talk, the woman went to call for the elevator, but the husband stayed behind for a quick thank you for Shockney. "We've been married 18 years and I've never had oral sex," he said. "Now I know we will, because she wrote it down."

TIPS ➢ ➢ ➢

1. Just because you're on hiatus from sex, don't forget to be affectionate with your wife.
2. Water-based personal lubricants, sold at drugstores everywhere, are a breast cancer patient's (and her husband's) best friend.
3. If your wife's white blood cell counts are really low during chemo, she might want to ask the doctor or a nurse whether it would be wise to engage in sexual intercourse. "Thrusting along the walls of the vagina could potentially introduce an infection," notes Philadelphia breast radiation oncologist Marisa Weiss, M.D. That could be problematic if your wife's immune system is weakened.

➢ BONUS TIP

If you fell out of the habit of sex during the chemo months and aren't sure how to recommence now that treatment is over, think back to courtship days, suggests Mary Hughes, a nurse at M.D. Anderson Cancer Center in Houston. Surprise your wife with a romantic Saturday night out. Who knows, maybe you'll get lucky!

Infusion Confusion

A guide for the bewildered spouse

If "cancer" is one of the scariest words in the medical lexicon, "chemotherapy" is surely among the most intimidating terms in the vocabulary of cancer. Chemotherapy may be a certainty because of tumor size or cancer spread. In some patients, the treatment is proposed before surgery as a way to shrink the tumor. In others, chemo may be up for debate. But in all cases, it is a matter of odds—will your wife gain enough of a survival benefit to justify months of chemotherapy drugs?

The breast cancer husband can be his wife's sounding board and confidant as she makes her choices, roles he already may have played in the surgeon's office. He can be the second set of ears at her appointments, if that is a job he handles well. He can continue to remind his wife of facts and figures she did not process, and keep track of the questions that she wants to pose—as well as the answers she might forget in her cancer-imposed state of stress. Because there's a lot she might not absorb. "A patient comes in with the notion that the cancer is early-stage," says oncologist Fred Smith, M.D., who practices in Chevy Chase, Maryland, "and then I say, 'Well, I think you need chemotherapy.' BOOM. The patient shuts off and doesn't hear 'to help improve the odds of staying well.'" Above all, the breast cancer husband is the one who can hold his wife and tell her he loves her more than ever. And there's never been a better time to show your affection. Chemo can provoke enough anxiety to make a breast cancer patient—and her husband—feel as if they could each use a Valium the size of a hubcap.

THE NATURE OF CHEMO

Chemotherapy is "adjuvant" or "systemic" therapy. If you're like me, you probably aren't sure exactly what these terms mean. Adjuvant means "giving help or aid." In cancer lingo, the word is used to refer to therapies that supplement surgery. Systemic means that the treatment covers the entire body, from head to toe.

And what is chemo, exactly? Powerful drugs are administered intravenously and/or orally; these substances seek and destroy cancer cells. Chemotherapy may play a small role in reducing the patient's risk of a local recurrence—another tumor in the breast. But its primary function is to wipe out microscopic breast cancer cells that may have migrated from the breast to other parts of the body, where they could eventually cause metastatic disease—breast cancer that has spread to the bone or to organs like the lungs, the liver, or the brain. Once metastatic disease is confirmed, a doctor's mission is to control symptoms and enable the patient to live with the disease, as a diabetic lives with her diabetes. (See the chapter titled Mysteries of Metastatic Disease on page 246 for more information.)

Unfortunately, chemotherapy drugs are indiscriminate killers. Sure, they can wipe out cancer cells. But they also mow down other rapidly growing cells throughout the body: white blood cells, hair follicles, and many other innocent bystanders. As the weeks and months of chemo go by, your wife will suffer a range of side effects, from mild to debilitating. Her immune system will be weakened. Injections of a drug like Neupogen may be necessary to keep her white blood count high enough to withstand the next round of chemo. Or she may need Procrit to boost her red blood cells. A woman might even need to be hospitalized if her white blood count drops too low and she develops a high fever—although that's not a common occurrence. But antibiotics might be necessary if she's ill and her white blood cells are in short supply.

Depending on the mix of drugs in the chemotherapy infusion, your wife will most likely lose her hair, and maybe even her eyebrows and eyelashes (see the chapter titled Hair Today, Gone Tomorrow on page 225 for a husband's guide to his wife's hair loss). She might also lose her fingernails, her energy, her period if she is pre- or peri-menopausal, her libido, her vibrant skin tone, the sparkle in her eye, her ability to concentrate and remember stuff (aka "chemo brain"). And she may lose her lunch as well (although researchers have made great strides in developing better meds to help control the nausea). So there's some good news. Otherwise—how do I put it nicely?—chemo sucks.

Or, as Dr. Smith explains, "Medicine in general is supposed to make you feel better. We have learned over time that surgery has short-term pain attached to it, but the goal is cure. All of a sudden, we offer something that's going to make you sick." Yup, that's chemo. Worst of all, your wife has to keep coming back for more. And more. And more.

FINDING AN ONCOLOGIST

The medical oncologist will be a key figure in your wife's current and future care. This physician is the all-around cancer expert on the team: the doctor tuned in to the subtleties of a patient's tumor makeup and the appropriate chemotherapy and hormonal treatments. And this is the doctor who would treat metastatic disease as well, should that ever come to pass. You and your wife will most likely refer to this doctor as simply "the oncologist," not "the medical oncologist." But the title "medical oncologist" does differentiate this doc from surgical oncologists (surgeons who specialize in treating cancer) and radiation oncologists (physicians who treat cancer patients with radiation therapy).

Not every breast cancer patient is a candidate for chemotherapy; it is estimated that about half of the 200,000-plus women diagnosed each year in the United States undergo chemo. But every breast cancer patient should see an oncologist to rule chemo in or out, and to discuss hormonal therapies—pills like tamoxifen and Arimidex—that might be able to reduce her chance of recurrence in the future.

An oncologist who treats many breast cancer patients will have the same advantage as a surgeon who is a breast specialist, or who does a great deal of breast surgery: heightened expertise gained from experience. Your wife will want the doctor to know the latest protocols and trial data, and to have treated enough breast cancer patients to have an instinctual feeling about what drugs could work well for her. "There are oncologists who treat everything," says Patricia Ganz, M.D., an oncologist who is a professor of health services and medicine at the UCLA Schools of Medicine and Public Health. "Lung, colon, breast cancer. That may be a fine physician to see, but getting a second opinion from a breast oncologist at a cancer center is advisable. Breast cancer is all that I do. Sometimes there are nuanced decisions that a general oncologist just doesn't understand. And breast cancer is much more nuanced than lung or colon cancer. The standard therapies are more narrow for those cancers."

So mistakes can be made, in both chemotherapy and post-chemo treatments. A few days before I spoke with Dr. Ganz, she had seen a pre-

---

DON'T PUT OFF UNTIL TOMORROW WHAT YOU CAN DO TODAY

Your wife may not want to start looking for an oncologist until after her surgery. You may share her view—let's finish up with the surgery before thinking about the next stage.

While you may want to put off the hunt for an oncologist—one less thing to do right now!—your wife will divest herself of a large amount of stress once she has chosen her docs and knows what her treatments will be. And so will you. So while she's running to see surgeons and scheduling surgery, she should be visiting oncologists, too—or at least be setting up appointments—because many oncologists are extremely busy. The oncologist's input could be critical at this point; some patients now receive chemotherapy to shrink the tumor before surgery. A tag team approach may work in the scheduling derby—she might be pursuing appointments with some docs, you with others. I still remember the morning of September 11, 2001. I was on hold with an oncologist's office when a colleague dashed into my office and said, "A plane just hit the World Trade Center." I'm a reporter by trade, but I knew where my responsibilities lay: "Sorry, I can't even think about that—I'm on cancer duty."

menopausal breast cancer patient whose oncologist recommended anastrazole (aka Arimidex), a drug taken after chemotherapy to reduce estrogen production in the adrenal gland. That sounds like a reasonable recommendation, because estrogen can feed certain tumors. But anastrazole only works in *post*menopausal women whose ovaries no longer produce estrogen. "That's completely inappropriate," Dr. Ganz says of prescribing anastrazole for a premenopausal woman.

The surgeon who treats your wife will surely be able to give her the names of oncologists who work largely or exclusively with breast cancer patients. So will family members, friends, or colleagues who've been through treatment. Unless your wife has complete and utter faith in the first oncologist she meets, you might urge that she visit a different oncologist for a second opinion. And perhaps even a third. Two experts can have differing opinions—a reminder that medicine is indeed an art as well as a science. There may be just small variations in their recommendations, or there may be significant differences. "Most oncologists are happy to have a second person collaborating," says Dr. Ganz. If they're not, your wife might ask herself if she would be happier with another doctor.

But there's a limit to how many oncologists your wife may want to see. "If you get more than three or four opinions, the patient may get confused," warns oncologist Adam Brufsky, M.D., codirector of the Magee-Womens Breast Cancer Program in Pittsburgh. If two or three doctors tell her roughly the same thing, he says, then she can feel confident that she's on the right track.

The oncologist your wife selects should be accessible as well as knowledgable, because that's who she'll call to report any unusual symptoms once treatment is over. "You want a doctor who will treat you like a person and explain things to you," says Dr. Brufsky. "And you can tell pretty quickly if that's the case."

Like any cancer doc, the oncologist should fill your wife with a spirit of optimism and hope whenever possible. And like any doctor, the oncologist should take the time to answer your wife's questions. If a question concerns a choice of chemotherapy regimens, the answer shouldn't be "that's what I do for all of my patients," suggests oncologist Victor Vogel, M.D., director of the

Magee/University of Pittsburgh Cancer Institute Breast Cancer Prevention Program. I was incredulous: "Would an oncologist really say such a thing?" His reply: "I've heard of doctors saying, 'This is the way we always do it.' Or, 'Don't question me. I'm the oncologist. Just do what I say.' Or, 'This is the way we're going to do it. If you don't like this, go somewhere else.'"

Which is exactly what you should do if an oncologist makes such statements.

My wife and I were fortunate. We met with three oncologists, and each one was smart, compassionate, and patient with our bumbling questions. So how did we choose?

Location, location, location. My wife's breast surgeon told us, all things being equal, to think about the location of the oncologist's office as one factor. I thought she was joking at first. But in hindsight, I'd say she was absolutely right. Your wife will make many, many visits to the oncologist's office. She will go for blood count checks, infusions, and follow-ups. You may be driving her there and waiting with her, or dashing from work to meet her there, or picking her up at the end of treatment and taking her home. (Or friends and other family members may be taking this job.) At any rate, if your wife has met with several oncologists and has good feelings about each one, and feels that their level of expertise is comparable, there's nothing wrong with figuring that a 15-minute drive from home or from her office is better than a 40-minute drive.

Take a look at the chemo room, too. That's where your wife will sit for the infusion of chemotherapy drugs. If the room has an ambience that is in any way appealing or at least not off-putting, that's another plus for that oncologist.

But a choice based on location or atmosphere is not always possible. My wife and I are fortunate to live in a part of the country where oncologists who specialize in breast cancer are plentiful. In other areas, the wisest choice may be to visit a university breast cancer center, even if it means a long commute.

THE CHEMO EQUATION

According to current National Institutes of Health guidelines, chemotherapy is recommended for a woman age 70 and under if she has a cancerous breast tumor 1 centimeter or larger, with or without lymph node involvement. But that's a guideline, not a law. A woman might have a tumor as large as 2 or 3 centimeters with "well-differentiated" cancer cells, says Robert Siegel, M.D., who is director of hematology and oncology at George Washington University Medical Faculty Associates in Washington, D.C. (That's a fancy way of saying that the tumor cells closely resemble normal breast cells and are slow to spread.) If the tumor is sensitive to hormonal therapy, the patient might be able to skip chemo without compromising her chances for long-term survival.

It's a matter of looking at the risks and benefits, and coming to a decision that makes the most sense for an individual patient.

The benefit of chemotherapy is quite clear. Every breast cancer patient has a certain risk of the cancer coming back. Chemotherapy will slice that risk by about one-third. That's the relative survival benefit of chemo.

What your wife needs to hear is the *absolute* survival benefit in her case. First, you need to know her risk of recurrence—it might be 10 percent (that is, 1 of 10 women with her cancer profile will have a recurrence). Or it might be 50 percent, if the tumor is large and the cancer is invasive. To find out how she will benefit from chemotherapy, multiply 30 percent times her personal risk and subtract the result from her personal risk. A 10 percent risk would drop to 7 percent. A 50 percent risk would drop more sharply, to 35 percent. "The bigger or more aggressive your cancer," says James Goodwin, M.D., chief medical director for geriatric medicine at the University of Texas Medical Branch at Galveston, "the bigger the underlying risk of dying, and the bigger the potential absolute benefit of chemotherapy."

You won't have to do the math. The oncologist will tell your wife the absolute survival benefit. (Just remember that "absolute" doesn't mean that your wife absolutely won't have a recurrence of cancer.)

Then the doctor must weigh the risks for a patient. If your wife is in excellent health, she can most likely handle the rigors of chemo. If she has heart disease, has had a heart attack, or has other serious medical problems, chemotherapy could pose a threat to her overall well-being. "There's no size that fits all," Dr. Siegel says, "because different patients have different needs."

DECISIONS, DECISIONS

How does the chemo equation play out on the marital front? "Ultimately, chemotherapy is the woman's choice," emphasizes Claudine Isaacs, M.D., an oncologist at Georgetown University's Lombardi Cancer Center in Washington, D.C. "Is it worth it to her? When you talk about a 3 percent benefit, no two patients react the same. A husband and wife might react differently. I imagine these things test marriages just like other strains."

In the end, the wife is the patient. The husband is not. In some cases, Dr. Isaacs sees a clear split: The patient wants one thing; the husband is not supportive. Sometimes the husband favors a more aggressive approach. Dr. Isaacs says, "I've had a couple of patients tell me, 'I wouldn't do this, but my husband really wants me to.'"

Conversely, the woman may be the one who wants chemotherapy, much to her husband's dismay. Nurse care coordinator Anne O'Connor, who also works at the Lombardi Cancer Center, remembers a husband and wife with young kids; the oncologist told them that chemotherapy would increase her odds of survival by an additional 10 percent. The husband thought that wasn't enough to justify 6 months of chemo. The wife said, "I want to live to see my children graduate from college." She was ready to suffer for her 10 percent benefit—and her husband came to accept her decision.

In another scenario, the patient may want chemotherapy and the doctor may not think it is indicated. "If it is a 'gray zone' and the patient feels strongly about receiving chemo, I will give it if they understand the risks to their health," says oncologist Sharon Giordano, M.D., an assistant professor in the department of breast oncology at the University of Texas M.D. Anderson Cancer Center in Houston. "If chemo is clearly not indicated or I think it is unsafe to give, I won't give it. If the patient and doctor reach a total impasse, which is unusual, then often it is best for the patient to switch doctors."

Or a doctor may think that chemo is a good idea and the patient may not. In that particular case, a husband might be stuck in the middle. He can ask his wife: "Would you have any regrets if you did not have chemo and you later developed metastatic disease?" But he cannot make the decision for his wife.

Then there are women who decline chemo and prefer alternative treatments instead. That can be a distressing situation for a husband (and for a doctor, too). A patient can't be arrested for refusing chemo, or dragged into the doctor's office like a naughty child and forced to take the drugs. All a husband can do is tell his wife that medical science knows that chemotherapy can be an effective tool in the fight against breast cancer. And that he's afraid if she doesn't try it, he may lose her.

THE REGIMEN

A few years ago, pretty much every breast cancer patient was treated with the same prescribed chemo regimen. Today, oncologists refer to the "alphabet soup" of chemo drugs that can be mixed in various ways and administered at various intervals. Why more than one? Drug combos are more effective cancer-busters than a solo actor. But the different chemo recipes haven't been tested against one another; that's why there isn't a consensus as to which combination works best.

Your wife will probably have four, six, or eight rounds of treatment with drugs like Adriamycin or Cytoxan or Taxol or Taxotere, administered at set intervals—every week or two or three. In some instances, the patient has a series of chemo treatments prior to surgery to shrink the tumor, and then

---

QUESTIONS FOR THE NURSE

Nurse practitioner Patricia Clark suggests that at your wife's initial visit with the oncologist, she spend at least a few minutes talking to the oncology nurse in the office. Among the questions to pose:

1. What is a typical treatment like?
2. Are appointments for the treatment room usually running late or on time?
3. Is there a time of day or day of the week when the treatment room won't be very busy?
4. What is the plan for anti-nausea medications?
5. If anti-nausea plan A doesn't work, what's plan B?
6. What if I call after a chemo round and say my anti-nausea or pain medications aren't working? How long will it take to get a new prescription?
7. Can you make changes in prescriptions without talking to the doctor?

GUY TALK

"Stefanie's done 6 months of chemo twice. The first thing to remember is that chemo is the good guy. Sometimes it seems otherwise. Visualize it blasting all those cancer cells."

—CHRIS SPIELMAN, 38
Columbus, Ohio

another round post-surgery. Presurgery chemo will give a clear indication if the drugs are working, notes Dr. Giordano. If the tumor shrinks enough, a patient may be eligible for a lumpectomy instead of a mastectomy. "But there still isn't any proof that survival rates are better," Dr. Giordano says of presurgery chemo. Some surgeons believe it is appropriate to perform a lumpectomy in such cases. Others aren't sure. "I still recommend a mastectomy if the lesion is very large," says Frederick Greene, M.D., of the Carolinas Medical Center in Charlotte. Why? "You don't know where the margins are, or if cancer cells would be left behind," he explains.

Dose-dense chemo is a new way of delivering the drugs—every 2 weeks instead of every 3, with additional Neupogen shots to keep a patient's white blood cell count from dropping. "It's quite controversial," says Dr. Giordano. Certain chemo drugs may be more effective with an accelerated time frame—"but it hasn't been sorted out."

The doctor's chemo prescription for your wife will be based upon the nature of the tumor, your wife's age, and other data. At a presurgery appointment, the oncologist will look at information about the cancer from the biopsy: the estimated size of the tumor (or tumors), estrogen or progesterone receptor status, the invasiveness of the cancer, family history, and so on. That will enable the doctor to make an initial recommendation about chemotherapy. The recommendation will be fine-tuned after surgery, when the final pathology report reveals more information about your wife's tumor and lymph nodes.

THE CATCH

The trouble with all this talk of the "absolute survival benefit" conferred by chemotherapy is that there is still no guarantee that your wife will actually do better if she undergoes months of chemo than if she passes on the treatment altogether.

Basically, there are three possible outcomes. Some women do indeed benefit from chemotherapy. They avoid or delay a recurrence or metastasis and add years to their lives. Some women could skip chemo and it wouldn't matter. They'd be just fine anyway, with or without it. And some women will go through chemotherapy and will still suffer a recurrence or metastasis at some point, and may eventually die of the disease. Maybe chemo will buy them some time, but maybe it won't.

So your wife must make a leap of faith. I hate to use that cliché, but that's how my wife's oncologist put it, and that's what it is—a leap of faith; hoping that if you take chemotherapy, it will help you, but knowing that it may not. Doctors also like to call chemotherapy an "insurance policy" against recurrence. That made my wife laugh. It's not really an insurance policy if your wife is one of the women who experiences a recurrence anyway. Just another of cancer's not-so-little ironies.

Older women have another point to ponder. There is little data regarding the effectiveness of chemotherapy on breast cancer patients over age 70. But you don't want a doctor who dismisses the possibility of chemo for older patients. "There may be subsets of women over 70 for whom chemo works, and others for whom it is harmful," Dr. Goodwin says. What you want is an oncologist who will say to a breast cancer patient, regardless of her age, "I feel in my gut that given what your tumor looks like, you would benefit from chemotherapy." Or the opposite—that chemo would not make a significant difference in her prognosis.

Then your wife must make a decision that she can live with and that will give her hope for a long and healthy life.

As she wrestles with her choices, you can do something for her that no doctor can. "Women are just frightened out of their minds that chemo will change them permanently," says Dr. Brufsky. "The important thing for the husband is to tell her, 'Yes, you are still the same person inside, and you will be the same person when it's all over.'"

TIPS ➢ ➢ ➢

1. Carolyn Hendricks, M.D., an oncologist who practices in Montgomery County, Maryland, and primarily treats breast cancer patients, likes to review the recommended chemo regimen and frequency of treatments at the end of an appointment. If your doctor doesn't make this a habit, go ahead and ask for a recap—and write down the doctor's recommendation.
2. Ask the oncologist about a port or catheter as a delivery mechanism for chemo drugs—a way to spare the chemical assault on your wife's veins. The port is implanted surgically in the chest. The catheter is easier to implant (and remove). In the doctor's office, it can be inserted under the skin just beneath the collarbone. But unlike the port, the catheter must be flushed daily with heparin solution and have a dressing change once or twice a week.
3. Find out the name of the person at your oncologist's office who is on call evenings and weekends, or if the doctor is out of town. And ask if an oncology nurse from the office is the contact for questions during the day. You are likely to get an answer more quickly from the nurse—some doctors can't get to their phone calls until evening.

➢ BONUS TIP

When chemo is done, your wife may be a candidate for hormonal therapy. The oncologist will discuss the potential benefit of medications like tamoxifen or anastrazole (Arimidex), taken for 5 years to reduce the odds of a recurrence. The newest pill in the medicine cabinet, letrozole, is taken after the 5-year regimen of tamoxifen or Arimidex and may offer 5 additional years of protection.

Coping with Chemo

A caregiver's tool kit includes medical reminders, hard candy, and back rubs

I vividly remember Marsha's first chemo treatment. On a mild Friday afternoon in November, she picked me up at work. We rode in nervous silence to the doctor's office. She sat in a tan Naugahyde chair in the crowded chemo room. An exceedingly nice oncology nurse pumped her full of anti-nausea medications. Then the chemotherapy infusion began. Her drug regimen was CAF—Cytoxan, Adriamycin, and 5-fluorouracil (aka 5-FU—yup, really).

I don't think we spent more than 2 hours in the room, because these particular drugs don't take too long to administer.

I had brought along a book on tape and a Walkman. Marsha wasn't interested in listening. I also had purchased Garrison Keillor's *Pretty Good Joke Book* to cut the tension. I told her one of Keillor's pretty good jokes. At the time, it didn't seem all that funny. So I thought up my own pretty bad joke: A chemo room looks a lot like a beauty parlor—comfy chairs, candy at the receptionist's desk, old copies of *People* magazine. Only nobody ever comes out with their hair looking better than when they went in. Marsha rolled her eyes and laughed. She was thinking the same thing.

The oncology nurse gave Marsha a flurry of prescriptions—for anti-nausea pills and for the so-called magic mouthwash that would prevent chemo-induced mouth sores. We stopped at a pharmacy, and then we went home. Marsha felt a little unsettled, but she didn't feel terrible. She had her appetite. We ate dinner with the kids—a kind friend had dropped off a casserole and salad. We watched TV. We went to bed. All the while, I felt as if I were in the countdown before a blizzard or a hurricane—when the weather forecaster predicts a storm is coming, but you don't know when it's going to hit.

Meanwhile, my head was spinning with all the theories about the nature of chemo passed on from well-meaning friends. The first chemo is the worst because your wife is so anxious. No, the second is the worst because she's let her guard down. No, it just gets worse and worse each time.

In Marsha's case, the storm broke 24 hours after the first infusion. Around 4:00 P.M. on Saturday, she began feeling queasy and dizzy and just generally bad.

At the time, I was surprised by the delay. I mentioned this to one of the oncologists I interviewed for the book.

She asked sharply, "Did they not tell you?" (that it sometimes takes a day for the drugs to kick in).

You know, I bet they did. And I bet it was just one of the many nuggets of information that my shell-shocked wife and I didn't quite process.

WHAT TO EXPECT

That's what your wife wants to know. You do, too.

Expect the unexpected. No two people go through chemotherapy exactly the same way. The first infusion might well be the worst. It's certainly the one that causes the most anxiety. "You can talk to a patient until you're blue in the face and walk them through it," says Patricia Clark, a nurse practitioner at the University of Michigan, Ann Arbor, and an oncology nurse for 21 years. "But you have no idea until you go through it. When you come back for the second, you may be a little more relaxed." But overall, she says, "each treatment is unique." For Marsha, the third wasn't too bad at all, the fourth was a grind, the fifth, and the sixth—I don't even want to talk about them. That's because there is one thing you can usually count on: The toll that the chemo drugs take is cumulative. That is, your wife will most likely feel (and look) worse and worse as time goes by.

Chemotherapy defies the rules of everyday life—the craving we all have for order and predictability. Your wife can certainly ask about scheduling appointments to fit into her routine. But severe side effects or a low white blood cell count could mean delays. When oncologist Patricia Ganz, M.D., who teaches health services and medicine at UCLA, sees a breast cancer husband whip out his Palm organizer to enter the chemo appointments, she warns, "You'd better not do that. You need to be flexible."

Yes, very flexible.

"At the very beginning, they assigned us a time for chemo, a regular slot," David Kupfer says, thinking back to the time when his girlfriend, Cathy Hainer, was diagnosed with stage IV disease. "I remember Cathy told me, 'Thursday at 1:00 P.M.' I got out my Week-At-A-Glance. And she said, 'David, this isn't the kind of thing you need to check your schedule about. You're going to be there.'"

At least, I hope you're going to be there. Setting foot in a chemo room takes a lot of guts. *Here I am, now give me the drugs that make me feel like crap!* Having a companion for moral support is a boon. Husbands can fit the bill, as long as they don't faint at the sight of needles or grow antsy in a clinical setting. Some husbands come to every session. Other couples work out different arrangements. "I went to the first chemo," says Bostonian Jonathan Davis, 46. But his wife, Michele, wanted him to be able to work, and her friends were "banging down the door" to go with her. Plus, her mother and sister wanted to lend a hand. "She worked it out and made a schedule," Jonathan says.

What if your wife insists she can handle chemo by herself? If she really means it, respect her wishes. Some women truly don't want their husbands to be with them in the chemo room. But your wife might be grateful if you come anyway. And she might not have a choice. Many clinics insist that patients bring a companion to ensure that they make it home safely after the infusion. Your wife may feel groggy from the anti-nausea drugs—some of them can act as a sedative. Ativan, for example, quells nausea as well as anxiety (now there's a welcome bonus) but can cause brief short-term memory loss.

No matter what drugs are in her chemo cocktail, your wife should have a volunteer chauffeur on call.

PRE-CHEMO MAINTENANCE

The husband can play a helpful role before chemotherapy even begins. While cancer docs worry about her cancer, they might forget to mention that she should tend to general health matters in the weeks before her first chemo. "She is going into a phase where everything revolves around chemo," explains Patricia Clark, the oncology nurse. "Anything your wife does on an annual basis, if it's about time for the appointment, move it up." (Or if the timing isn't critical, postpone it until after chemo.) And who better to remind her than you?

Here's the short list:

The annual physical. Depending on how long chemo lasts, your wife might figure this one can slide, since doctors are poking and prodding her with great regularity.

Teeth cleaning. A pre-chemo cleaning is a good idea. Everyone's mouth is full of bacteria, and a cleaning might release some of the bacteria into the bloodstream, which is what you don't want to have happen during chemotherapy. "If the white blood cell count is low, there is no ammunition to fight infection," Clark explains—and adds, "Sorry for the wartime metaphors but, in some ways, this is a war."

Flu shot. If it's the season, you and your wife should get one.

Pap test. This isn't an especially comfortable procedure to begin with, and the vaginal dryness that chemo can cause won't help matters.

A manicure and pedicure—the bonus extra. Fingernail and toenail work might not be the best idea during chemo, when your wife wants to avoid potential infections. "It just makes you feel better," laughs Stacey Boyle of her foot pampering. "You're on chemo and you're ugly, but your toes look nice."

DOUBLE-CHECKING THE DOSE

In 1994, a Boston breast cancer patient died because she was given the wrong dosage of chemo drugs. She was on a high-dose chemotherapy regimen. An oncology fellow misinterpreted the protocols and called for four times the prescribed amount; other doctors signed off on the order.

In another more recent chemo scandal, a Midwestern pharmacist was diluting the drugs to pad his pocketbook.

Carla Greenberg remembers her last treatment, coming home and feeling glad it was over, and then getting a call from the oncologist's office—"they forgot to give me one of the drugs. I had to come back."

Luckily, these errors are rare. And since the overdose tragedy that cost the woman her life, more checks have been built into the system to prevent such mistakes.

"First of all, the doctor checks the dosage calculations," says oncologist Victor Vogel, M.D., who directs the Magee/University of Pittsburgh Cancer Institute Breast Cancer Prevention Program. "A collaborative practice nurse who works with each oncologist checks as well. The dosage calculation is given to the pharmacist, who prepares the medication and checks the calculations for the third time. And finally, the medicine is given to the chemotherapy nurse, who administers the treatment. She also checks the name, the drug, the dose, everything about it, to make sure it's done correctly."

That's four separate sets of eyes. Still, some breast cancer patients feel the need to check for themselves.

"The thought that you are going to take this stuff that can affect your immune system, make you lose your hair, your menses, has got to be frightening," says oncologist Fred Smith, M.D., who practices in Chevy Chase, Maryland. "It takes a huge leap of faith, and a lot of solid information, and then a tremendous amount of courage. If, in that process, it helps put the patient at ease to know exactly the dose and the mix, I think that should be offered and respected."

So if your wife is so inclined, she should go ahead and double-check. Or she might delegate the job to you. "I know couples where the husband has done that," says oncologist Adam Brufsky, M.D. "Look, if it makes you feel better, that's okay."

Ask the oncologist what dose of each drug is being prescribed for your wife, how the dose was calculated, and under what circumstances—weight loss, weight gain—the dose should be changed. Write down the information. And verify it each time. If your wife is getting IV chemotherapy, look at the IV bag to make sure her name is on it. "I

THOUGHTS ON FOOD

Even if 100 friends are cooking dinners for your family during chemo, sometimes you'll bear the responsibility for preparing meals. And you won't really know how to cater to your wife's chemo-charged taste buds. Chemo leaves many women with what they describe as an "icky" metallic taste in the mouth. A food your wife has always liked might suddenly be intolerable. A food she enjoyed last night might taste awful in the morning. In fact, all food might seem loathsome. She might develop an aversion to meat, or salt, or sweets. So what's a breast cancer husband to do? I'm glad you asked.

Hydration. Very, very, very important. In the first day or two after a chemo treatment, your wife might not feel like eating a thing. That's okay, as long as she drinks. But even water might be hard to get down. Tap water and bottled spring water all have a taste that typically doesn't even register as a taste, except to chemo patients. Distilled water is the taste-free water that chemo patients might guzzle if other waters don't sit well, says nutritionist Lynda McIntire of Potomac, Maryland, who advises breast cancer patients. If your wife has a soft spot for ginger ale, tell her to drink up. Even if the soda doesn't contain enough ginger to quell nausea (sprinkle some in, if you want a higher ginger count), many people think of it as a "comfort drink." The gentle carbonation might settle her stomach, and there's no caffeine to stir things up. However, Jeffrey Rosenbaum, D.D.S., my diligent dentist, cautions that sipping sugary soda through a straw all day is not the best thing for the teeth, especially at a time when the patient may be letting dental hygiene slide. Diet soda, anyone?

Hard candies. They can help your wife deal with the metallic taste chemo causes—especially candies with strong flavors, like lemon, coffee, or mint. When Gary Krimstein's wife, Becky, was feeling queasy, he ran out to the drugstore and bought every kind of candy on the shelf. Five years later, Becky still has a package of wintergreen Life Savers tucked away in a drawer—a made the infusion nurse show me the dosage every time and explain why I was getting that dosage," says Heidi LaFleche. "It was helpful to have my husband there as another pair of ears, to make sure it was the right amount."

---

minty-fresh symbol of her husband's devotion. (Dental warning: Again, Dr. Rosenbaum notes that sucking on sugary candies all day is an invitation for cavities; he proposes sugarless hard candies, although your wife's taste buds will most likely dictate her choice.)

Avoid favorites. If you're the one fixing meals after chemo, don't pamper your wife with her favorite dish. It sounds like a nice idea, but it could backfire. The food she's always enjoyed will then be linked in her brain with chemotherapy. Once chemo is over, the sight or smell or taste of that meal could prove intolerable.

Fix healthy meals. Women may think they'll lose weight during chemotherapy, with the nausea and taste bud alterations. In fact, chemotherapy patients typically put on pounds. They may be less active because chemo saps their energy. The push into menopause alters metabolism for the worse. Serving up high-calorie concoctions will only add to the problem.

Bland may be better. Particularly after the first go-round, when your wife's reaction to chemo is as yet unknown. "Sometimes, a simple scrambled egg and canned fruit can be very appealing," even if your wife wouldn't touch such a meal normally, says Melanie Polk, a registered dietitian and director of nutrition education at the American Institute for Cancer Research in Washington, D.C.

Don't take it personally, part I. The night of a treatment, I fell into the habit of fixing grilled breast of chicken, mashed potatoes, and a green vegetable. But after a few cycles of chemo, Marsha couldn't stand the thought of what seemed like comfort food. Sometimes, you just have to accept that "what you're trying to do isn't going to help that day," says Lita Smith, a nurse practitioner at the University of Michigan Comprehensive Cancer Center in Ann Arbor.

Don't take it personally, part II. Even the onions on your breath from lunch might bother your wife's chemo-compromised nostrils. Try a breath mint. And the next time you go out for a meal, hold the onions.

JOB LIST

If you're the kind of breast cancer husband who's looking for jobs to do, then chemo is cut out for you. For some chemotherapy drugs, a patient must take pre-medications. Offer to keep a checklist and issue reminders. You can also take charge of the prescriptions your wife needs to have filled after each session. And you can keep track of questions that come up between treatments. Make sure that your wife asks them when she goes in for the next infusion—or that you bring them up if the stress of chemo has her forgetting to inquire.

Marsha had complained to me of feeling flushed and woozy the second the IV started delivering meds to her. She figured that's just how it was. An oncology nurse asked how things were at the start of one session; I thought I'd mention Marsha's reactions. "She shouldn't be feeling that way," the nurse said. "Maybe it's the anti-nausea medication." She switched to another drug, and Marsha felt much less woozy during and immediately after her time in the chemo-room chair.

Your wife might appreciate a useful suggestion from Jean Lynn, an oncology nurse who is the program director for the Breast Care Center at George Washington University Medical Faculty Associates in Washington, D.C. The standard chemo routine is for the patient to have blood drawn for the all-important "counts," then wait for word from the lab. If the white blood cell count is too low, chemo will have to be delayed. "Have the counts done the day before you see the doctor," Lynn suggests. That means an extra trip to the doctor's office, but it eliminates the uncertainty on chemo day.

In the chemo room, you can offer moral support. Julian Trujillo, 72, of Ramona, California, would stand behind his wife, Evelyn, and put his hands on her shoulders while she was getting her infusion. Sometimes he would read psalms. "It was reassuring," says Evelyn, 69. "It was just wonderful, beautiful."

You can offer a sweater, too . . . or a shawl . . . or a blanket. Some chemo drugs are refrigerated and cause a chill when delivered into your wife's veins. Even fluids kept at room temperature are 20 degrees colder than body temperature, notes oncology nurse Patricia Clark. Remind your wife to dress in layers, and offer to bring an extra wrap. Some women like to bring a comfortable pillow as well.

A breast cancer husband makes a fine gofer in the chemo room. Tethered to a pole from which her IV bags are hung, your wife may crave a drink of water, a hard candy, a magazine to leaf through. Or she may need help flagging down an oncology nurse for a question, since oncology nurses tend to be a tad overworked.

The husband can be an advocate for his wife, too. At chemo number four, Marsha needed a Neupogen shot to boost her white blood cell count before she could get the infusion. From the grimace on her face at past shots (and from her very vocal complaints), I knew that the shot can sting like a swarm of hornets. That particular afternoon, Marsha told the nurse who was tending to her that she just couldn't stand to endure a Neupogen injection.

"Suit yourself," the nurse said, and walked away.

So there Marsha was, all tethered up and no way to get chemo. And there I was, not quite sure what to do. "I'm going to talk to Fran*," I said—referring to a good-hearted nurse who previously had treated Marsha. I explained the problem to Fran who kindly came and sat by Marsha. The two of them talked for a few minutes, and Fran persuaded her to take the shot. I'm still not sure if Marsha was inclined to thank me.

HOW WILL SHE FEEL?

Probably lousy, but not necessarily. Various chemo drugs produce different reactions. And different women have different reactions.

Some patients sail through chemo with minimal nausea and malaise. Stacey Boyle still chuckles at the comment of a woman she met at a breast cancer survivor gathering: "Girlfriend, I went to work at Kentucky Fried Chicken every day I was on chemo, and then I'd tell my husband, 'Bring me some water, I'm thirsty.'"

Stacey wasn't so lucky. Diagnosed at age 35 with advanced breast cancer—a 5-centimeter tumor, two positive lymph nodes—she had her first chemo on Halloween. "I told them I wanted to go trick or treating and have some fun with my daughter, and the nurse said, 'You'll be fine.'" That night, Stacey says, "I was so bloody sick, I was projectile vomiting; it was real, real bad." Her husband, Michael, called the doctor, who had to come up with emergency prescriptions. "I just couldn't keep anything down for 4 days. They had to give the anti-nausea medicine to me in suppository form. It was really unpleasant." The doctor told her that once in a while he meets patients who have an extraordinarily hard time with chemo, "and you're one of them."

Most women fall somewhere in between daily stints at KFC and projectile vomiting. The current round of anti-nausea medications really works wonders for many patients. But that's not to say they're feeling good. And most husbands (like me) wonder, *what does it really feel like?*

After that first chemo, Marsha said she felt as if she'd just ridden the world's tallest, fastest, upside-down roller coaster . . . and she's a woman who gets dizzy on a merry-go-round.

"Is it like the flu?" Chris Rippie prompts his wife, Debra Wood, who was his fiancée when she was diagnosed. "I don't like being nauseous," Debra answers. "And this was to the next degree of nausea. The nausea was unbearable. Oooh, I just wanted to lie in bed and stay there in that fetal position. You're not doing chemo justice if you tell someone it's like the flu."

HELPFUL HUSBANDS

Short of filling the anti-nausea prescriptions, can the breast cancer husband help combat post-chemo ills?

"He tried to fix it, and there was nothing he could do to fix it," says Susan Taylor of her husband Vern's response. Nothing helped her except for moaning. But the sound of her moaning made Vern want to tend to her even more. And Susan would say, "Oh, shut up and let me moan." If he couldn't stand it, she says with a laugh, she'd tell him to leave the room. The point is that sometimes your job is just to commiserate.

You might give your wife comfort by telling her to imagine the chemo drugs as powerful allies in the fight against cancer—which they are. But that's not for everyone. The word "infusion" drove Allen Salzberg crazy. "They put a needle in my wife and found a vein and probed around so they could put in some really strong chemicals that on a higher level would probably kill her," says the 50-year-old New Yorker. "And the word for that is 'infusion.'"

My wife and I had a similar reaction to chemotherapy. Yes, we get it, it's *therapy*. But frankly, we liked the nickname that comic Julia Sweeney gave to chemotherapy in her cancer memoir, *God Says Ha!* She called it "Drano."

Whatever your feelings about chemo, you should be at your wife's beck and call. "I did whatever Lois asked," says Dale Hazel. "If she got hungry for something, I got it. If she wasn't up to doing much, I would tuck her into bed."

A little gesture can mean a lot. "He rubbed my back and that was good," says Linda Ellerbee, remembering her chemo months—and how her companion, Rolfe Tessem, held her constantly.

Keep an eye on your wife's teeth, suggests Jeffrey Rosenbaum, D.D.S., who practices in Washington, D.C., and often treats patients going through chemotherapy. If your wife vomits after chemo or has frequent reflux, Dr. Rosenbaum suggests that she (or you) ask the dentist for a prescription toothpaste with extra fluoride, or for a fluoride mouthwash to protect her teeth from the acid. Chemo patients also may suffer from a lack of saliva—another reason for a fluoride mouthwash. It'll help rinse the teeth in lieu of natural saliva. In addition, dry mouth can lead to a yeast infection in the mouth or just make the patient's mouth feel sore. Your wife's dentist should be able to recommend an artificial saliva product as well as a rinse to anesthetize the tissue and make the mouth more comfortable.

Mind-body therapies might make chemotherapy more bearable. There are no guarantees, but some women swear that they feel better if they avail themselves of acupuncture, yoga, meditation, massage, or guided imagery (the latter involves listening to an audiotape that takes your mind on a vacation from cancer and chemo). There are plenty of tapes for sale. A husband with a soothing voice can even make a tape for his wife. You can find guidance in books like *30 Scripts for Relaxation Imagery & Inner Healing* by Julie Lusk and *Rituals of Healing: Using Imagery for Health and Wellness* by Jeanne Achterberg and Barbara Dossey. Or try improvising: You're walking on the beach, feeling the sand in your toes, hearing the birds calling. "If she's afraid of water, that's no good," says nurse Patricia Clark with a chuckle. But she has seen guided imagery work. "For people who do guided imagery regularly, it can actually lower the heartbeat and respiration rate, make you just generally more relaxed." And that might make chemo a little more tolerable.

Massages made Lois Hazel feel better—but Dale wasn't sure they could afford regular sessions: "That's like $70 a pop. And her income was greatly reduced; she was on disability. We couldn't afford 70 bucks a week for a massage. But, we couldn't afford not to. My attitude was, 'We've been behind before. We'll get caught up.' But I didn't say that to her. I said, 'You want the massage, we'll get it.' We couldn't spend our money in any better way."

WORKING DURING CHEMO

If your wife is employed, she will have to make a decision about her work schedule: Will she keep going to the office, scale back, or take a medical leave?

Each woman does what feels right to her. And the husband's job is to support her.

"I didn't work," says Cynthia Duncan. "I did not go to my job from the day of diagnosis in August until March." She had a stressful job handling huge movements of money for a trust department. "I decided I didn't need that. My job was to take care of me."

Her husband, Richard, was fine with that. He thought that getting the stress out of her life could only help in her battle with cancer.

Other husbands think work is a cure for what ails a chemo patient. One fellow told me, "I can't understand why my wife is on disability. She's not disabled. The data points show that women who work do better during chemo. If it were me, I'd be working."

I had to bite my tongue to keep from saying, "But it's *not* you."

Truthfully, I can't say that I was a model husband either. I had the opposite problem. Marsha, who teaches high school, wanted to work. She felt that cancer had stripped her of so much already—flesh, hair, a sense of well-being. She didn't want to let it take away every element of her identity. Plus, if she were to stay home, she'd just end up feeling sorry for herself. She wanted to keep her routine going. She wanted to be productive and busy. And she didn't want to spend every minute of the day thinking about how lousy chemo was making her feel. Many breast cancer patients share her views.

But then I saw Marsha drag herself to school on days when I thought she'd be better off at home, napping and watching guilty-pleasure TV. And I felt as if I were failing as a husband. Shouldn't I insist that she stay home? That she take it easy just 1 or 2 more days after her chemo infusion before heading back to the fray? I would beg her to give herself a little more time off.

What I learned was that I could say what I had to say—and I did, because I'm not shy. Then I would follow the breast cancer husband's credo: "Shut up and listen." Months later, when I described my dilemma to oncological social workers, they suggested that I could have tried to be a problem solver. Instead of just saying, "Marsha, you're crazy. Stay home. What are you trying to prove?" maybe I could have been a little more diplomatic and constructive: "Honey, can you think of a way you'd be able to take an extra day off if you feel that you need to?"

But in the end, Marsha solved her own problem. The offer of a student teacher came up. She was reluctant at first—too much work training a novice. Finally, she took the offer, and as the chemo side effects grew more and more unpleasant, she was deeply grateful to have someone to help grade papers and teach a few of her classes.

Carol Stevenson was another chemo trouper. Working as a financial manager for the Defense Department during her treatment, she remembers how she'd "drag my weary body into work" even though her husband, Phil Gay, thought she might be better off taking a sick day. On one particular day, her blood pressure was so low that every time she stood up, she'd practically pass out. A coworker escorted her to the office clinic and called her husband to come and get her. "He was kind enough not to say, 'I told you so,'" Carol recalls.

How did he resist the temptation?

"I learned a long time ago," Phil says, "there's a time to be a smartass and a time to keep your mouth shut."

COUNTING DOWN

Odds are that one of you will be counting off the months, weeks, days, hours, minutes, and seconds until that last chemo visit. Your wife might take heart from checking each chemo off on the calendar. Katy Kelly remembers x-ing off each day as if she were a prisoner, waiting to be sprung.

Then again, your wife might be ticked off if you keep saying, as I did, "Two down, four to go; three down, three to go . . . " "That doesn't make me feel any better," Marsha would say. I thought about her response. If I were going to be mowed down by a truck six times, would I take comfort from the fact that only two hit-and-runs awaited? Nope. So I shut up, although I was secretly thrilled to see the end growing near.

Your wife might also decide that she just can't deal with one more chemo. "One day I refused to go," says Lois Hazel. She told her husband, Dale, that she was sick and tired of being sick. He let her get it all out, and then said, "You're going to your chemo, aren't you?"

And Lois said, "Yes, but I don't want to." Dale hugged her. And then she went.

For some women, a hug might not be enough. Lita Smith, a nurse practitioner at the University of Michigan Comprehensive Cancer Center in Ann Arbor, remembers how one husband's words helped his wife, who had suffered from horrible nausea and vomiting after her first three chemo infusions. Her husband said, "Honey, I love you. I understand this is horrible, but we don't want to look back and say, 'Shoulda, coulda, woulda.'" At first she cried, but when the time came for chemo number four, she was feeling a little better and said, "Okay, let's just do it."

In the meantime, you can try to relieve the monotony any way you can. There's always sex, if your wife is feeling up to it (see the chapter titled The Intimate Details on page 171). And there's travel. It's risky, as Carla and Dick Greenberg discovered when they had to turn back at the airport because Carla wasn't up to a flight from Washington, D.C., to San Francisco. But Marjorie Turgel made it all the way to the Arctic Circle. She and her husband, Ray, had booked a summer cruise months before. Then Marjorie was diagnosed with breast cancer. In between chemos three and four, she and Ray

GUY TALK

"Reading aloud is a wonderful way to be with someone who is undergoing chemo. I'd read to my wife from Heidegger. When she got nauseated, all I had to do was stop reading—that was our joke."

—JAMES GOODWIN, 58
Galveston, Texas, describing the role played by the ponderous German philosopher in the chemo room

flew off to Scandinavia and boarded the ship. Her oncologist gave her the names of hospitals in major cities nearby, just in case, and the names of oncologists in the area as well. She did just fine.

That's a bit daring. A "chemo treat" can be a bit less ambitious—a trip to a favorite museum, a movie or play or concert, a dinner out. Just having something on the calendar to look forward to every couple of weeks can help. But check with your wife before making reservations. "I know one couple where the husband wanted to go to restaurants," says nurse Patricia Clark. "And she'd look at him like, 'You're nuts, I'm going to vomit!'" So maybe fancy restaurants aren't the best idea. You get the picture.

And actually, Hester Hill Schnipper did get the picture. When the oncological social worker from Concord, Massachusetts, was going through chemotherapy for her breast cancer, she visited an art gallery with her husband and fell in love with a painting of two trees, whose deep, intertwined roots kept them standing tall in the face of a fierce windstorm. In the middle of chemotherapy, she felt like one of those trees. When she finished her last chemo treatment and came home, her husband had a surprise. The painting was waiting for her.

TIPS ➢ ➢ ➢

1. According to studies, women who exercise during chemotherapy may feel better than those who don't. Invite your wife on a relaxed 15- to 30-minute walk. It can't hurt, and the calorie-burning can help fight another chemo side effect: weight gain.
2. If your wife needs Neupogen shots at home to boost her white blood cells, she might do it herself, or she might ask for your aid. Jonathan Davis says EMLA cream, a prescription topical anesthetic, was a salvation for his needle-sensitive wife. Applied an hour before an injection, the cream numbed his wife so the prick didn't make her wince (though the injection did).
3. Don't be a pigheaded "I-can-do-it-all-myself" breast cancer husband. Accept offers from others to watch the kids, fill in on carpool duty, and provide dinner. And if your family has any particular food dislikes, speak up or be prepared to eat cold cereal that night. If no one's offering, go ahead and ask. "People want to help," says nurse practitioner Lita Smith, of the University of Michigan Comprehensive Cancer Center in Ann Arbor. "But sometimes they don't know how."

➢ BONUS TIP

If your wife is prone to motion sickness, she may be more likely to suffer nausea or to vomit from chemotherapy drugs. Encourage her to share that fact with the oncologist or oncology nurse, who might prescribe anti-nausea meds accordingly. You also might stop by the drugstore and buy her the Sea-Band, a bracelet that applies pressure to the point on the wrist that controls queasiness, according to acupuncture principles. Or buy fresh ginger at the supermarket, slice it, and tell her to take a deep whiff. Some women have success with such tactics. If they work for your wife, you'll be her hero!

Unconventional Cancer Care

How couples navigate complementary and alternative therapies

Tooling around the Web one night, you stumble upon a miraculous cure for cancer—shark cartilage capsules. No, I'm not making this up. Promoters claim that the substance cuts off the blood supply of tumors.

A neighbor swears that guzzling wheat grass juice made her breast cancer disappear, and offers to whip up a batch for your wife. Yum, yum or dumb, dumb?

A coworker who had breast cancer tells you that acupuncture was the only way she could conquer her post-chemo nausea. "You've just got to make an appointment for your wife," she urges. You can't help but think, "If I don't, what kind of husband am I?"

Welcome to the world of complementary and alternative medicine—also known as CAM. And it is indeed a world unto itself, where healers tout the benefits of all sorts of unconventional therapies for cancer patients. Some of these treatments are intended to help patients cope with the assaults of surgery, chemotherapy, and radiation. Others are billed as ways to lick the cancer itself. The treatments are sometimes paired with the usual medical treatments (that would make them complementary) and sometimes proposed in lieu of conventional care (then they're alternative).

You and your wife may not be CAM-compatible, and that's perfectly okay. Many patients don't pursue such therapies and do just fine. But your wife may well be interested in experimenting. A study published in the *Journal of Clinical Oncology* in July 2000 polled 453 cancer patients and found that nearly 7 out of 10 had tried at least one CAM option. If either (or both) of you is intrigued, the best advice is to proceed carefully. There are indeed potential benefits to unconventional cancer care. But there are potential dangers as well.

WHAT DO WE KNOW?

You've no doubt heard of some of the more popular CAM therapies—yoga, meditation, massage. But you may not be sure how they help a cancer patient. (Actually, the goal of these practices is to reduce the stress caused by chemo and other treatments.) Others probably sound unfamiliar, like guided imagery (that's summoning up mental images to ward off worries or promote healing) and Reiki (a healer's hands direct your "universal life energy" to where it's needed). In addition, health stores and catalogs sell an array of anticancer pills and herbs.

But do the therapies really work?

In 1998, the National Cancer Institute established the Office of Cancer Complementary and Alternative Medicine to conduct studies and come up with answers. Overall, the office sounds a cautionary note: "While some scientific evidence exists regarding some CAM therapies, for most there are key questions that are yet to be answered through well-designed scientific studies—questions such as whether they are safe, and whether they work for the diseases or medical conditions for which they are used."

But there's always new research going on. One current study seeks to determine whether "shark cartilage extract may help shrink or slow the growth of colorectal cancer or breast cancer cells." Who knows, maybe the extract will become a respected part of the arsenal of treatments in years to come. Then again, it could turn out to be just another anticancer scam. One thing we do know: despite what the pro-shark-cartilage forces say, sharks *do* get cancer.

A cancer patient has to be careful when looking for the scoop on CAM. Information is plentiful. Reliable information—well, that's harder to come by.

Web sites are full of unsubstantiated claims. You can, for instance, still find online testimonials to the curative powers of laetrile, a compound derived from the pits of plants, even though a 1982 study sponsored by the National Cancer Institute found no evidence of lasting improvement in cancer patients treated with the substance.

For a sampling of current (and reliable) information from academic centers and cancer groups like the American Cancer Society, start by logging on to www.nlm.nih.gov/medlineplus/canceralternativetherapy.html. As always, breastcancer.org is a good source as well. Type in the name of a CAM therapy in the site's search window and see what comes up.

When I was curious about acupuncture, I visited breastcancer.org and learned about a study presented in 2000 at the San Antonio Breast Cancer Symposium. A group of 104 women were being treated with high-dose chemotherapy; all of them were given anti-nausea drugs. They were split into three groups: no acupuncture, minimal needling, and electro-acupuncture, which applies weak electrical currents to the needles. The women who had no acupuncture had a higher degree of nausea and vomiting. Regular acupuncture provided some relief. Electro-acupuncture gave a significant amount of relief. So there you have it—proof that needles can be helpful along with pills. That isn't to say every cancer patient will embrace the Chinese healing art (as I'll explain later on in the chapter).

AN ADVOCATE'S ADVICE

Even if you're a skeptic, you must respect the fact that CAM therapies are a beneficial tool for many breast cancer patients. Carole O'Toole of Kensington, Maryland, is living proof. Ten years ago, O'Toole was diagnosed with a 5-centimeter tumor and inflammatory breast cancer, the rare and rapidly spreading kind. She was 38 and the mother of a 2½-year-old daughter. The first surgeon she saw told her she had 18 months to live, no matter what she did. Needless to say, she found another doctor and endured a mastectomy, chemotherapy, radiation, and a bone marrow transplant in her battle against cancer.

Along the way, Carole turned to complementary therapies—"to alleviate some of the side effects, to boost energy and spirit, and to support me in my recovery." Before trying a treatment, she would do "exhaustive" research, and then talk with doctors, CAM experts, and breast cancer survivors. She admits there was a bit of trial and error in the process, but when she found a therapy that made her feel better, she went for it—because when you're fighting for your life, you need all the help you can get.

Some of her treatments might strike a skeptic as a tad offbeat. In energy work, for example, a healer places hands on or above a patient to channel "universal energy" that will aid in the healing process. For Carole, such treatments were a balm for body and mind.

Ten years after her diagnosis, she works as a cancer coach, helping women cope with the disease and all the decisions they must make. The advice she gives to her clients is good for husbands to hear: "I tell women, this is a time when you have to mother yourself as if you are your own sick child. And complementary therapies allow you to nurture yourself."

Want to learn more? Carole is the coauthor of a guide to complementary cancer treatments: *Healing Outside the Margins: The Survivor's Guide to Integrative Cancer Care.*

Looking back, Carole is grateful for the therapies that gave her strength—and is especially grateful for her husband's support. "He is the king of all pragmatists," she says. "He would not have gone with complementary therapies himself. But he never laughed at me when I told him what I was doing. His attitude was, whatever you need to help yourself heal."

FULL DISCLOSURE

Whatever complementary or alternative therapies your wife embraces, she should tell her doctor. The number one rule of pursuing CAM is to tell all. And I do mean *tell all.* She should share every CAM therapy she's contemplating with her regular cancer docs. (The only exceptions would be purely mental activities, such as meditation or journal writing.)

Has your wife visited a healer who gave her a list of herbs, beverages, or vitamins to ingest? She should bring the list to her next doctor's appointment. She also should mention her interest in treatments like acupuncture and massage. She might be taking a substance or undergoing a treatment that would

GUY TALK

"I'd feel impatient spending too much money on Chinese herbs and wheat grass, but I felt clear that my job was to be a support; and that meant if Cathy wanted wheat grass, it's her life and I'm not going to say, 'Don't buy it.'"

—DAVID KUPFER, 51
Arlington, Virginia, whose fiancée sought conventional and unconventional treatments

not marry well with surgery, chemotherapy, or radiation. "We don't know what interactions many herbs and such have with traditional treatment," explains Johns Hopkins nurse Lillie Shockney. "For example, taking shark cartilage before surgery can result in severe bleeding due to the effect it has on the vascular system."

If your wife is not inclined to discuss her CAM treatments with her cancer doctors, you can—and should—suggest that she do so. (Although you shouldn't tell without her consent.) Perhaps she is worried that her doctor won't be supportive. That could happen. But cancer doctors are often open-minded. "There are some people who need to feel they're taking a hand in their treatment," says Yale University clinical professor of surgery Sherwin Nuland, M.D., who is the author of *How We Live* and *How We Die*. "Many of these people like to go and see a homeopathic physician or a holistic medicine physician. One never stands in the way of that as long as that doesn't stand in the way of standard therapy."

Your wife will certainly be better off if a doctor reviews her proposed complementary treatments. When David Kupfer's fiancée, Cathy Hainer, wanted to drink wheat grass smoothies in her battle against stage IV breast cancer, hoping the preparation would strengthen her immune system and enable it to defeat the cancer, that was fine with her oncologist. Even though the American Cancer Society notes that "there have been no scientific studies in humans to support any of the claims made for wheat grass," wheat grass does not appear to pose any health risks. But Chinese tea earned a thumbs down. "If you don't know what's in the tea, I'd suggest you not take it," the doctor told her. "A lot of Chinese teas have estrogen, and estrogen can feed breast cancer." And what if your wife is seeing a CAM practitioner who insists that conventional treatments aren't the answer. "Be wary of anyone who says 'My way is the one way,'" says James Gordon, M.D., a Harvard-trained psychiatrist who directs the Center for Mind-Body Medicine in Washington, D.C.

NO GUILT

The number two rule of CAM is that a patient shouldn't beat herself up if the therapy doesn't work. Just as conventional treatments for cancer do not always keep the cancer from recurring, there is no guarantee that CAM therapies will produce the desired result—be it a boost in energy or a cure for the disease.

Consider the connection between the brain and the immune system. Medical researchers are currently studying the power of the mind. They are trying to determine whether positive or negative thoughts can have an impact on an individual's health. And there is certainly evidence that stress plays a role in one's health. But that's a long way from saying that a woman's state of mind can prevent or cure breast cancer. "The fact of the matter is that there may be psychological factors in breast cancer," says Dr. Nuland. "But right now we don't know what they are. And there isn't a shred of evidence that bad thoughts give you cancer or that good thoughts cure you. The only thing good thoughts do is make it possible to live a somewhat happier life during this awful time."

In his book *How We Live,* Dr. Nuland sums up the dilemma by recounting the case of Sharon Fisher, diagnosed with breast cancer at age 35 while 6 months pregnant with her second child. Based on her 7.6-centimeter tumor and positive lymph nodes, Dr. Nuland believed she had only a 1 in 4 chance of living 5 years. When he wrote the book, Fisher was a 12-year survivor—and a great believer in "keep[ing] yourself positive" with meditation, imaging, and other "nonmedical" practices.

"She is certainly right about optimism's effect on the quality of life . . . and she may also be right about its not-infrequent effect on longevity," Dr. Nuland wrote. "My clinical observation leaves me with conflicting beliefs. For every

Sharon Fisher, I have known a dead optimist." (A new study raises similar doubts about the power of a positive outlook. Researchers in Australia followed 179 lung cancer patients. Within 5 years, 96 percent of them had died regardless of whether they were optimistic or pessimistic about their chances for survival.)

If a patient tries CAM therapies with great faith in their power, and the therapies do not work, what is she to think? Dr. Gordon advises people to pursue CAM therapies with an open mind and heart. But if things don't go the way you hope, he stresses, don't fall into the trap of thinking, "I have done something wrong." Radiation oncologist Irene Gage, M.D., who practices at Sibley Memorial Hospital in Washington, D.C., has stronger words: "I worry that this is just another way to make a woman feel guilty about something she has no control over."

Yet it is precisely the cancer patient's loss of control that makes CAM appealing. "They feel they are doing something on their own behalf," says Mary Johnson, a nursing professor at Minnesota's Saint Olaf College and a CAM advocate. One of her dear friends was diagnosed with breast cancer and pursued traditional treatments as well as untraditional therapies. "She embraced all of the herbs, she followed a macrobiotic diet, she exercised, meditated, and received massages and healing touch," Johnson says. And her husband made her a daily cabbage juice drink, a popular CAM anticancer concoction. "It was something he could do for her that was loving and caring," Johnson says.

None of the treatments—conventional or complementary—saved Johnson's friend. But when it became apparent that her death was imminent, she did not feel that she had failed. "She felt she had fought the good fight," Johnson reflects. "In the end, the outcome is in the hands of the Lord."

COUPLE CONUNDRUMS

You and your wife won't necessarily agree about CAM. That could be a small problem—or a large one.

Let's talk about the less critical situation first.

I was the guy whose colleague raved about the powers of acupuncture. I'm certainly open to CAM therapies, so I shared the story with my practical-minded Yankee wife. She wasn't especially interested. But I prevailed. Setting

Marsha up with an acupuncturist seemed the perfect way for a husband to "fix" something about cancer. My wife's oncologist was supportive, giving us the name of an acupuncturist who worked with breast cancer patients.

I made an appointment for the day after a chemo treatment. Over the course of an hour, the kindly acupuncturist stuck all sorts of needles into Marsha's "energy points." (No, it didn't hurt, she reports.) Then he eased the needles out and sent her home with a magnet for added relief. The bill came to $100, which was not reimbursed by our insurer.

That night, Marsha was on her knees, retching into the toilet. Coincidentally, she had begun taking antibiotics the day before because of an angry red welt on her arm that raised fears of infection, and she has a history of

CAN PRAYER CURE CANCER?

A number of mind-body disciples believe that the answer to that highly charged question is yes: Patients who pray to be healed—and even patients whom others pray for—will fare better or live longer. Such thoughts are reflected in the mainstream as well. According to a *Newsweek* magazine poll, 4 out of 5 Americans are confident that praying for a patient ups the chance of recovery.

A skeptic might say, "Prove it." For years, researchers have been trying to do just that. In a frequently cited 1988 study, Randolph Byrd, M.D., a cardiologist at the University of California at San Francisco Medical Center, assigned 393 heart attack patients to two groups: standard medical care and standard medical care plus prayer on their behalf by "participating Christians." The patients in the latter group did not know they were the subject of prayers. Dr. Byrd found that the prayed-for patients had fewer instances of congestive heart failure, didn't need as many antibiotics, and did not need as much help breathing as those in the control group. "These data suggest that intercessory prayer to the Judeo-Christian God has a beneficial therapeutic effect in patients admitted to a coronary care unit," Dr. Byrd concluded.

But efforts to replicate the study's results have not been successful. What's more, a report published in 2000 by the Hastings Center in Garrison, New York, which researches bioethical issues, pointed out significant strong reactions to antibiotics. While the antibiotics most likely brought on the vomiting, Marsha was not inclined to return to the acupuncturist for a second go-round. You know, the power of association . . .

So I didn't fix anything. And I learned a $100 lesson about complementary therapies: They're not for everyone. "It never hurts for a husband to suggest anything, recognizing that the person may decline," says Morry Edwards, Ph.D., a Michigan psychologist who works with cancer patients and is the author of *MindBody Cancer Wellness: A Self-Help Stress Management Manual.*

A more difficult husbandly dilemma arises when a breast cancer patient wants to embrace alternative therapies instead of conventional treatments.

---

problems in studying "prayer as therapy." Investigators cannot know with certainty that one group of patients is being prayed for and the other isn't. There's no way to create a uniform prayer for all individuals of all religious backgrounds. And, of course, there is really no way to prove beyond the shadow of a doubt that prayer will protect you from the shadow of death. "Petitionary prayer may make people feel better," says Richard Sloan, Ph.D, a professor of behavioral medicine in the department of psychiatry at Columbia University and a sharp critic of claims about the healing power of prayer. "But there is no medical evidence that it is beneficial."

And if a true believer prays, and the prayers are not answered, then what? "That's the problem," Dr. Sloan says.

But there is another benefit to prayer, and it has nothing to do with the potential for a cure. "We pray from the heart," says Cynthia Duncan, diagnosed with breast cancer at age 46. "We talk to God as if He were our friend, and just say what's in our hearts. One night, I was really sick from chemo, and I asked my husband Richard, 'Is it wrong to pray to God not to feel sick?'"

Her husband answered, "Why don't you pray that God will give you the strength to deal with whatever comes?"

"Just doing that," Cynthia recalls, "made me feel better." And that's an irrefutable testimony to the power of prayer.

In theory, the husband should support his alternative-leaning wife. But keeping silent could be torturous if her decisions might endanger her life. One oncologist told me of a breast cancer patient who has been applying a black herbal salve to her breast, hoping the salve will dissolve the tumor. Months have gone by. The tumor hasn't gone away. The patient's breast has burns from the salve. The husband sits by his wife at appointments with a stricken look on his face.

Lillie Shockney suggests that such a husband might say to his wife: "From the research I've been doing for you on the Internet and in talking with cancer centers, I've learned there is no scientific proof that these remedies work. It scares me to think we might embark on a treatment that won't help and that might even do harm, and I don't want to lose you. I know having surgery and chemo and radiation may seem scary, but it would be a lot scarier for me to think about living without you at my side, because you made a decision to go with a treatment that isn't helpful."

It may take more than just one speech.

On the day of her breast cancer diagnosis 2 years ago, Laurie Ferreri had a previously scheduled appointment with a naturopath—an individual trained to use "non-invasive natural medicine" like herbology and biofeedback. At the time, Laurie was a true believer. Her husband, Jim Finkelstein, came along. He was a true unbeliever.

"The naturopath was a quack, a charlatan," Jim says. "She had Laurie questioning whether she should receive traditional medical treatment at a time when she was most vulnerable. I know Laurie has great respect for alternative medicine, but this woman was telling my wife not to get conventional treatment. I knew that if Laurie didn't get conventional treatment, there'd be only one outcome."

Jim tried to keep from exploding in the naturopath's office. He remembers thinking, "If I do anything other than sit here and be quiet, if I'm overly critical, the crisis will deepen."

Laurie grins, "Yeah, but you were exuding anger, and I'm sure your eyes were rolling back in your head when she gave you a lecture about modern medicine."

They left the appointment with a $150 bill for the visit and $400 worth of supplements.

Even though Jim's eyes had indeed rolled back in his head (and probably out the door), he took it slowly. "The challenge," he says, "was to find a way to help Laurie make a decision that would incorporate her beliefs." That meant locating an oncologist who was open to working with complementary practitioners. And it meant raising questions about alternative and complementary therapies. Jim's main question: "Where's the research?"

Often, there wasn't any.

"Whatever Jim did, it was the right thing," Laurie says in retrospect. "He stated his opinion, he showed me how upset he was, he didn't push it too far, and he made me realize that everything I do should be based on a good rational decision—and on research. If it weren't for Jim, I probably would be down that alternative route."

Instead, Laurie opted for traditional treatments—presurgery chemo, a bilateral mastectomy, more chemotherapy, and, finally, radiation. Whenever she could, she incorporated complementary therapies along the way. For example, her naturopath endorsed megadoses of vitamin A to promote healing after surgery, and Laurie followed that advice. That is, until she began complaining of joint pains, and her doctor mentioned that too much Vitamin A can cause . . . joint pains. "I hope to God that's what it is," Laurie says, although in the end it appeared that chemo was the culprit.

The Washington, D.C., couple can now joke about the hell they've been through. "This really cut into my golf," Jim, 51, complains in mock seriousness. "I'm taking my vitamin A now," Laurie, 54, teases back, popping a pill. (She's kidding, of course.) Jim and Laurie share an affectionate laugh—and you don't need a scientific study to know that laughter is good for the body, good for the soul.

TIPS ➢ ➢ ➢

1. Encourage your wife to talk to her cancer docs about any vitamins, herbal remedies, or other substances she's taking on the advice of a complementary or alternative healer.
2. Beware of Internet quacks. Web sites prey on vulnerable patients, hawking untested creams and pills as cures for cancer, and spinning tales of miracle cures—but failing to provide valid research to back up their claims.
3. James Gordon, M.D., the Harvard-trained psychiatrist who directs the Center for Mind-Body Medicine in Washington, D.C., is a fan of dancing for the sheer pleasure of it, of keeping a journal ("it provides companionship, release, insight, especially if you write fast and get over the idea that your mother will read it"), of meditation, and of good old-fashioned exercise.

➢ BONUS TIP

Nursing instructor Mary Johnson highly recommends the joys of hand and foot massage. She suggests 5 minutes (minimum) per appendage, with music playing so the husband-masseur can block out distractions. A firm touch, she says, will help prevent a case of the tickles.

Hair Today, Gone Tomorrow

Helping your wife handle her hair loss

The shedding of hair is a sign that the chemo is doing its job. But try telling that to your wife. Weeks before her first treatment, Marsha couldn't stop talking about the hair, the hair, the hair.

I understand that no one wants to go bald, not even temporarily. But I couldn't quite understand why Marsha had such a hard time accepting the inevitable fact that her hair would fall out. Not only was she upset about losing her hair, but she worried about its rate of regrowth as well. She would ask me, "Do you know how long it will take before my hair grows back to the length it is now?"

I didn't have a clue.

But Marsha had already done the math. At the rate her hair grew each month, it would take 2 years for her light brown locks to once again fall just below her chin.

Sometimes I wanted to yell, "Enough already!"—especially when Marsha was raising these concerns with her oncologist. At the time, I was thinking like a typical guy. I felt she was fixating on what seemed to me a trivial issue, instead of asking about the bigger, more important aspects of her treatment. Yes, the hair will go, I wanted to say, but it will grow back. And there's nothing you can do about it, so try to make your peace with it and move on.

In her desperation, Marsha thought there was actually something she could do to ward off her hair loss. A well-meaning friend told Marsha that an Israeli doctor had invented a method to prevent hair loss during chemotherapy—a "cold cap" that chills the hair follicles and thus sets up a frigid barrier, keeping the chemo drugs from reaching the follicles and knocking them out. Since I'm the Internet researcher in the family, I googled around and found the magic cap.

Marsha's oncologist knew just what it was when we brought the printouts to our next appointment. He had, as it turns out, written a paper about the potential benefits of such a device back in 1983, because, as he wrote, "Alopecia [the medical term for baldness] is a striking reminder of the patient's diagnosis and the effects of therapy." But over the years, he had come to see that the cap didn't deliver on its promise. So he told us, "I don't think it works."

There's also a remote possibility that cancer cells lurking in hair follicles might survive if chemo doesn't reach them. And since the goal of chemo is to knock out all of the cancer cells in your body, leaving any behind would defeat the purpose of the treatment. In spite of all this, the oncologist took pity on my desperate wife. "If you wish," he said, "I can fashion you a cap."

Marsha and I were both deeply touched. But she didn't want him to make a cap that probably wouldn't work—or worse, that could allow cancer cells to remain intact. At that moment, Marsha made her peace with her impending hair loss.

THE BALD TRUTH

After talking to dozens of women, I have come to understand that for many of them the unkindest cut of all, as it were, is the loss of their locks. Husbands—be they bald, balding, or hirsute—need to let them mourn the loss.

Think of where your wife is at this point in her treatment. She's heard the chilling news that she has breast cancer. She has most likely gone through surgery and lost a piece of her breast, or perhaps the whole thing, or even the matched set. She's been told that chemotherapy is necessary to stop cancer cells from dividing in her body. But chemo has a similar effect on other rapidly growing normal cells—including hair cells. Not every chemo cocktail causes complete hair loss, but if the potent drug Adriamycin is in the mix, your wife's crowning glory will almost surely be a victim. Chemo could also wipe out her eyebrows, eyelashes, armpit hair, pubic hair, arm and leg hair.

So your wife will be a bald lady. Bald is usually not beautiful when it comes to women. And when you see a bald woman, you can almost bet that she's a cancer patient on chemo. So there's a double whammy: Your wife won't look her best, and everyone will know she's dealing with cancer.

To my amazement, many women have told me that losing a breast is not as difficult as losing their hair. A loose-fitting blouse can conceal the loss of a breast. But the bald head is such a public symbol of everything that's wrong, and her bald head will be staring her right in the face every time she looks in the mirror.

A CLOSE SHAVE

When your wife is facing chemo baldness, you might trot out the old sports maxim: The best defense is a good offense.

Cancer takes away control. A preemptive shave gives your wife back a bit of control. Instead of waiting for the inevitable, she's the one who decides when to go for the Demi Moore "G.I. Jane" look. But she does have to make the decision early on. Mike Malone recalls how the shaving of his fiancée's head was more of an "emptive" strike, since her hair was already on its way out. From the date of the first chemo, your wife has 10 to 12 days before her hair starts coming out in clumps. Within 48 hours after the shedding begins, the hair is usually gone.

Some women do it themselves. "My husband was making pancakes," says Joan*, 52. "I went to the bathroom, shaved my head with a Lady Gillette, came down, and said, 'Well, how do I look?'" Her husband spun around, took in her bald head, and didn't miss a beat: "You look beautiful."

Good answer!

But don't overdo it. "If you go too far overboard," says oncological social worker Hester Hill Schnipper, "it doesn't sound true." She thinks that many women just want to hear five simple words: "You look beautiful to me."

GUY TALK

"She asked me to shave her head. I thought I'd just go ahead and shave it. But it brought home a flood of emotions. Every emotion I had came out."

—KEN PRUITT, 46
Port St. Lucie, Florida

Husbands can assist in the shave if they wish. Jeffrey Berger, the always-prepared lawyer from Chevy Chase, Maryland, tried to make it fun, or at least less traumatic, for his wife. He wore an open-necked shirt for the occasion, like a hip European hair stylist, put on cool music, and took an electric shaver to his wife's curly red locks. They both had a good laugh over her visit to Salon Jeffrey.

On a family trip to the Appalachians in North Carolina, Aileen Pruitt, 42, was already down to a quarter-inch cut, but the stubble was bothering her tender scalp. So she asked her husband, Florida state senator Ken Pruitt, for relief. He lathered up her head and, with the razor Aileen used for her legs, whisked away the itchy remnants. "Did you cry?" I asked. "Oh yeah," he says. "It was a shaky razor." (Perhaps that's why hair professionals recommend an electric trimmer for the job, especially if your wife has already begun chemo. You don't want to risk any nicks if her infection-fighting white blood cells are on the low side.)

Lili Romero-DeSimone, 33, said goodbye to her long blond hair during a head-shaving party at her Alexandria, Virginia, home. Her husband, Steve Romero, got a buzz cut in solidarity. She told him to dare not go any further or "you're going to look like Uncle Fester."

It's your call, husbands. I haven't yet met a wife who ordered her husband to have a sympathy shave. But those guys who went all the way were glad they did.

Vern Taylor, 52, of Winnipeg, took a razor to his white hair when his wife was diagnosed with breast cancer in 1998. But his reason for doing so went beyond a show of support.

"When my wife and I first met with the surgeon, one question we asked was, 'Whom do you tell?'

"It was her advice that you tell everyone." Vern was surprised, because in his mind, cancer is a private medical condition, and a breast "is a somewhat private part."

But then he thought about it . . . and decided the surgeon was right. "I should tell everyone, let them know breast cancer really affects people, and more research ought to be done. People out there need to know."

A physical therapist who co-owns a medical device company, Vern figured that a shiny pate would be a good conversation starter, and he was right. People would say to him, "Whoa, you shaved your head. That's radical. What happened?"

When he would tell them, they, in turn, would share their moving stories about how breast cancer had touched their lives as well.

There is one thing to be careful of, however, when you join your spouse in baldness. If the two of you suddenly go hairless, and you have young children, tell them not to worry—nobody's going to mow down their hair in the middle of the night.

WIGGING OUT

As you and your wife sit in the waiting rooms of breast cancer docs, you'll undoubtedly come across colorful catalogs featuring wigs and scarves and hats for the chemo patient. The problem with these catalogs is that the women modeling this cancer headgear are fashion-model gorgeous. They could be wearing garbage can lids or string mops upon their heads, and they'd still look dazzling.

What's more, a wig is not a perfect solution. We guys might not know if a woman's hair isn't her own, but the female sex is adept at sniffing out wigs. "It doesn't matter how expensive it is," one breast cancer survivor says. "Even if I'm sitting a few rows behind someone in the theater, I can tell."

Your wife should not begin her wig shopping by looking in the Yellow Pages under "W." Your average wig shop is not prepared for cancer patients, and your average cancer patient is not prepared for a wig shop. "I went with this misconceived notion," says Lili Romero-DeSimone, who visited a neighborhood establishment. "I thought I'd make it fun, buy three wigs—blond, red, and black, like *Charlie's Angels*. I wasn't going to do this thing like, 'Make it look like my hair and pretend I don't have cancer.'" But in the wig store, women wearing lab coats, as if they were doctors, told her there would be a $5 fee for every wig she tried on. They told her the fee would be waived if she

---

GETTING WIGGY WITH IT

My wife did not ask me to shave my head or hers. That was a relief, because I didn't think I would have had the courage for either course of action. She didn't take me to the wig shop for the first visit, either. She preferred a female friend, and that was understandable. But she did invite me to come to the wig shop to advise her as they styled and fitted her new hair, and to hold her hand while a wig shop employee gave her the closest trim she'd ever had.

We sat in a small private alcove in the back of the busy store. An older woman with a Swiss accent cut Marsha's hair into a spiky helmet that was quite the hip 'do. The hair stylist saved the longest swatches of hair to make fake bangs for a headband (which Marsha never wore). Then she took out an electric razor and gave Marsha a buzz cut.

Now, you can do many things while you're sitting with your newly shorn wife in a quiet corner of a bustling wig shop. You can cry together, mourning the loss of her hair and fearing the future. Or you can hold each other quietly and whisper, "I love you."

Or you can goof around.

Do you blame me? There were boxes of wigs all around us. Dolly Parton wigs. Elvira, Mistress of the Dark, wigs. Wigs that transformed my wife into a Vegas blackjack dealer, a prim prison matron, a no-nonsense diner waitress. She indulged all my fantasies, and she still says to her friends, "I wonder what people thought when they heard a guy and his wife laughing hysterically in the wig shop."

I sort of wish she had gone for a cotton-candy-blond concoction. But the sensible brown wig that mimicked her usual style served her well. Sometimes the wig looked like a wig—maybe a touch too matronly, too stiff, too much like a helmet of hair.

But in the right light, with her wig upon her head, penciled-in eyebrows and well-applied makeup, Marsha looked like . . . Marsha. If I hadn't known that she was in the midst of chemotherapy, you could have fooled me.

bought the wig in question, but Lili wanted to try on a dozen wigs or more, if need be. She walked out "pissed off as could be, very bitter and upset."

Lili then went to a wig store that caters to cancer patients, and the staff treated her with sympathy and tenderness. (The oncologist's office usually keeps cards and brochures on hand for local shops that have years of experience drying the tears of their customers.) This time, her husband, Steve, came along, and when she hated the synthetic wigs, he encouraged her to go for the real thing. "I don't care what it costs," he said. "If it makes you happy, we'll work it out."

What made her happy was a $1,100 human-hair wig. "I didn't want to spend that kind of money on something as totally vain as hair," Lili says. Steve's attitude made the difference.

And the wig can make quite a difference in your wife's attitude. I paid a visit one morning to Amy of Denmark, a salon in Wheaton, Maryland, whose clientele includes many cancer patients. There I watched as Colene Frederick, 69, and her husband, Pete, 59, came in. He was pushing her in a wheelchair. She looked weary and worn, her white hair sparse because she'd already had chemotherapy.

"I didn't think losing my hair would be hard because I'm old," Colene said. "But it is."

The eponymous Amy Cordaro picked a few synthetic, silvery wigs in the $200 price range and let Colene try them on. She looked at herself in the mirror. In an instant, the weariness vanished; years fell off her face.

Colene asked Pete what he thought of one model.

"I don't care for that," he said. "It's not light enough."

She tried on another.

"I think it looks nice," Pete said.

Colene was soon admiring herself in the mirror and making goo-goo eyes at her husband. A few quick trims from Amy's deft scissors and the wig was ready to go home with Colene.

While Colene and Lili took their husbands along on the wig-shopping expedition, don't feel bad if your wife would rather go without you. She may prefer the company (and comments) of a female companion as she tries to decide whether to go wig wild or to find something that's a close cousin to her regular hairstyle. (Although that's not always possible. Some sort of bangs or feathering is needed in the front of the wig or else part of your wife's bald head might be visible. And really long wigs are not so easy to care for.)

If you are the one who accompanies your wife, you're inevitably going to be asked: "Do you like the way I look in this?" That is nearly as tricky a question as the dreaded "Honey, do I look fat in this dress?"

"If it's awful, you better say so," says Amy of Amy's.

"What husband wants his wife to have a buzzard wig?" chimes in Elan Bar-Haim, a stylist in the shop.

And you'd better tell the truth.

"Most women know if their husbands are lying," says Colene Frederick. "I can pretty much tell—they change the subject pretty fast."

A noncommittal grunt is just about as bad as a lie. Women don't care for that, says Hans Kalset, who has been fitting wigs on cancer patients for years at Lucien et Eivind in Washington, D.C. "I think they want him to say not 'Whatever' but 'Yes' or 'No.'"

Emotions run the gamut. Sometimes the woman and her husband cry. Sometimes Hans cries with them.

A husband who sees the wig for the first time may be taken aback. Hans has heard men say, "You told me there was a little change, but this is a lot of change."

And his wife will say, "Well, this is what I want."

"You feel how tense it is," Hans says. "He'll be putting pressure on her. But whatever she wants is how it should be."

THE PRICE OF LOOKING PRETTY

Wig experts say the same thing as prostheses dealers when asked about the price difference between models. "You can drive a VW or you can drive a Lamborghini," says Amy Cordaro. "You're still gonna get where you want to go."

But if you've got the cash, don't scrimp. A wig fashioned from luxuriant human hair can run well over $1,000. For that price, your wife gets hair that shines and swings. In the $500 price range, the hair might be a bit coarser. Some women prefer human hair, but others think it's creepy and are happy with synthetic. A nicely made synthetic wig will run $100 to $500. There are also real/synthetic blends, which hold the style well and look pretty real. By the way, if your wife goes synthetic, she'll need to doff her wig if she plans to do any cooking. The heat of an oven or stove won't be kind to a synthetic hairpiece. Better yet, you can do the cooking—or call a restaurant for home delivery.

If the cost of a wig is too much for your budget, call the American Cancer Society, which runs wig banks in various locales. A woman who cannot afford a wig (or does not want to shell out hundreds for a hairpiece she hopes she'll never have to wear once chemo is over) can borrow a wig.

Your health care plan may pay for some or all of the wig. But good luck in your quest. Different states have different rules. So do different health care plans. And your health care insurer may not know what you're talking about. You'll need a prescription from your wife's oncologist for a "cranial prosthesis due to chemotherapy-induced alopecia." Jim Finkelstein remembers being on the phone with a health care representative demanding coverage for a cranial prosthesis, and the poor woman on the other line had not a clue what he was talking about. Finally, she got it. "Oh, you mean a wig."

Yes, that would be it. A wig.

Perhaps your health care plan will inform you that, of course, the cost of a prosthetic device will be covered—as long as it is purchased from one of the authorized prosthetic device dealers that work with the plan. That's what Marsha's insurer told her. The problem is, prosthetic device dealers usually sell artificial limbs, not replacement hair.

You (or your wife, whoever is doing the calling) might face the old runaround. "Well, we don't make that decision," the clerk might say. "Your employer does." And your employer won't know what you're talking about. Whichever of you has the most patience for dealing with bureaucrats, take on the wig fight. It's probably the most absurd round of negotiating you will face when it comes to medical expenses, but at least you'll garner excellent material for the next dinner party you attend.

In our household, my wife did battle. And she did not stop fighting. She felt that if the plan covered prosthetic devices, and she had a prescription for such a device, well, then, show us the money.

At first, her insurer didn't agree. Then she wrote a letter.

Dear Appeals Unit,

I would like to appeal the rejected claim for my hair prosthesis due to chemotherapy-related alopecia. As stated in the members' benefits booklet on page 34, "Prosthetic and Orthopedic Devices" are covered under the Indemnity component. The booklet does not stipulate which prosthetic devices are covered; rather it is stated in a general way. Furthermore, on page 39 in the list of "What Is Not Covered," there is no reference whatsoever to excluding a hair prosthesis. In light of that, as well as the fact that there are state laws that mandate that hair prostheses for chemotherapy-related alopecia be partially reimbursable up to $350, this claim should be honored.

I would appreciate your reconsideration for this claim in a timely manner.

A minor miracle took place. They read the letter, and they caved! We got a check that covered a good chunk of Marsha's $600 wig.

WELCOME HOME!

The wig can come home with you that very first day if it's synthetic. Human-hair wigs may require dyeing and cutting—and a return visit for final fitting.

Your wife's new hair will live on a Styrofoam head (which helps to keep its shape). It'll require washing, even if it's synthetic. A human-hair wig will need to be styled after a shampoo, so your wife may want to turn to a wig expert. The wig store most likely provides this service for a fee—about $30; your wife's regular hair stylist may also be a capable wig washer/stylist.

Husbands sometimes pitch in with a synthetic wig. Any shampoo with conditioner will do, says Hans Kalset. He recommends lukewarm water, and treating the wig as if it were a fine garment. Then plop it on the mannequin head and it should dry nicely. Blow drying is not only unnecessary, but it could make the wig look as if it got a really bad perm.

As crazy as this may sound, you might want to name the wig. Lots of couples do. After all, it's a new member of the family. Stacy and Mike Malone of San Francisco, who got engaged shortly after she was diagnosed with breast cancer, went with the name "Lola," bestowed upon the wig by Mike's mom.

When Stacy and Mike were out and about, they had a secret code. Stacy might ask, "How's Lola looking tonight?" and Mike could offer his viewpoint.

Or if Lola was slightly askew, Mike could easily point that out. Best of all, neither of them had to utter the word they really couldn't stand: wig.

By the way, Lola wasn't an only child. Mike bought Stacy a purple wig. It turned out to be perfect for Halloween.

THE UNVEILING

Your wife may be timid about showing you her bald head. You may be afraid to look. Social worker Hester Hill Schnipper met one husband who didn't want to sleep in the same bed as his wife. She was furious at his seeming lack of interest. The truth was, he was nervous about seeing her nude noggin.

Some women wouldn't mind wearing a scarf in such a circumstance, says Schnipper. Others are offended by the thought of having to conceal their baldness. "If a husband says to me, 'I don't think I can handle her being bald,'" Schnipper asks if he's ever seen his wife's hairless head. She may keep her head covered with something at all times. Experiment a little, she advises. The wife might begin by going uncovered for a spell—not in bed for a sexual encounter, but just in the house, doing normal household things. This exposure may help the husband get a little more used to her baldness.

And really, it's not so terrible. Other couples make the adjustment just fine. Laurie Ferreri, 54, of Washington, D.C., remembers the night a hot flash hit when she was at a restaurant with her husband and friends. Off came her uncomfortable wig.

John Salamone, 35, of Alexandria, Virginia, made a sign that read "Bald is beautiful" and taped it to his wife's mirror.

Becky Krimstein went wigless in the house when she was going through chemo, and her husband, Gary, didn't mind at all. "The wig would be uncomfortable and itchy, and going bald was just free and natural," she says. Sinead O'Krimstein, as Gary sometimes called his shorn wife, would lie on the couch, bald and beleaguered from chemo, and he would rub her head. He discovered a birthmark he never knew she had: "That was cool." And she loved the massages: "It felt really good. He would say he was putting love in my hair. When it came back curly, he said he put too much love in there!"

NEW GROWTH

The months of chemo go by. Really, they do. And somehow your wife makes it to the last treatment. Her hair might even start growing back while chemo is still in progress. That doesn't mean the chemo isn't working, by the way.

In other cases, a few hairless weeks follow her final treatment before new growth begins to sprout. So be patient. When she says, "It's been 2 weeks and I don't see anything," look really hard and see if you can spot a patch of fuzz—like the first haze of green on the trees after a bleak winter.

Then comes this awkward period. Your wife has a crew-cut of sorts, but the wig still goes on because of pride and self-esteem and fear of what people will say and think. One day you may think your wife has enough hair to go wigless. And she won't. I've heard that story a few times, and I've lived through it, too.

When we went on vacation in late June, a couple of months after the end of Marsha's treatment, she had a short and spiky hairdo. I loved it. She wasn't sure how friends and family we'd be visiting would react. So the wig came on the trip, perched on its Styrofoam head in the trunk of our car.

We saw friends in New York. They thought she looked fine. We saw cousins in Vermont. They, too, thought she looked fine. By the time we got to Maine, I was fairly certain that the wig was never coming out of the trunk. The biggest test was the end of the trip, in Boston, when we'd see Marsha's mother and sisters. They're a tough crowd. I was afraid someone would say, "Marsha, you look like you have a bad crew-cut." I wanted to call ahead of time and say, "Tell Marsha she looks good." But I trusted in fate.

Everyone loved her hair.

Plus, as it went from buzz to bob, the hair was clearly curly. After chemo knocks out the hair follicles, new growth may have a different texture than the old hair. The color may be different, too. It could be gray (and it probably won't take hair dye too well at first). Or it could be a complete surprise. "No one takes you seriously when you look like Little Orphan Annie," laughs Carol Stevenson, who sported a post-chemo crop of red (and white and blond) ringlets before her fine, straight, blond hair returned.

Marsha's curls lasted a year. That's what most women told me about the duration of changes in their hair. Women who liked the curls joke about their "$100,000 perm." Those who didn't were relieved when their hair returned to its prior state.

Time will pass, and you'll almost forget that your wife was once a baldie. But you will have some memories. Some of them may be awful, and some of them won't.

Years after her chemo baldness, TV journalist Linda Ellerbee recalls how cold her hair-free pate would get on winter nights, and how her companion, Rolfe Tessem, would sleep with his hand cupped over her noggin to keep it warm. I can't think of a better picture of true love.

TIPS ➢➢➢

1. Make sure your wife goes to a wig shop that's accustomed to cancer patients. She'll get more TLC and she won't be hit with fees for trying on wigs.
2. Nurse and cancer survivor Lillie Shockney suggests a "coming out" party for your wife's pending hair loss. If you think she's up for it, get one of her close friends to do the planning with you. Invite her nearest and dearest buddies to come by and bring the gift of a head covering—anything from utilitarian hats and cashmere sleep caps to silly and outrageous headgear.
3. In many cities, the American Cancer Society runs wig banks that are chock full of loaner hair. For locations, go to www.cancer.org and select "prostheses and accessories" and type in your zip code.

➢ BONUS TIP

If your wife is feeling down about the way chemo has made her look, see if you can track down a local session of the "Look Good, Feel Better" program, offered by breast cancer centers working with the American Cancer Society. A makeup artist advises chemo patients on the art of camouflaging eyebrow and eyelash loss, how to wear scarves stylishly, and other cancer-relevant beauty tips. Visit www.lookgoodfeelbetter.org or contact a local breast cancer center for details.

Radiation: The Daily Dose

Side effects vary, but the need for support is constant

I was a radiation dropout.

Like many breast cancer husbands, I went with my wife to dozens of doctor's appointments and to most of her chemo sessions (her sister stood in for me once). I went to the initial appointment with the radiation oncologist and met the highly recommended Irene Gage, M.D., whose kind and knowledgeable manner inspires utter confidence. Marsha didn't feel the need to talk to any other radiation oncologists, especially after Dr. Gage said she had treated patients with bilateral breast cancer (which is what Marsha had). Plus, the good doctor practices at Sibley Memorial Hospital in Washington, D.C, which sits right on Marsha's commute to work.

When it was time to begin radiation, after the surgery and the many months of chemo, Marsha became a solo act. She felt okay going it alone, stopping by for her radiation rendezvous on the way home from the school where she teaches. And I felt relieved that I could return to a regular work schedule.

In that respect, I was a pretty typical male. Dr. Gage doesn't see a lot of husbands. "Some of them come to the first appointment, and I get a sense of how involved they are," she says. "A lot of times they can tell their wife is feeling fine and doing fine, and they feel comfortable, and she feels comfortable going it alone." Occasionally a husband comes to every single appointment, which may or may not be a blessing. "The wife might prefer some time by herself," says breast radiation oncologist Marisa Weiss, M.D., of Philadelphia. But there are husbands who never show up to meet the radiation oncologist. Ever. "Rightly or wrongly, I usually feel like that's a red flag on some level," says Dr. Gage.

Some of those solitary women tell her they feel so alone, as if no one is paying any attention, and they're still expected to make dinner each night, and they're really tired. Greg Passler, who took his wife to many of her treatments, remembers meeting a woman in her 60s whose biggest concern was finishing her radiation appointment on time so she could rush home to make her husband lunch. The Master of the House was sitting at home (at the kitchen table, no doubt) and would be ticked off if he didn't get his meal. I have a counterproposal for hubbies of this ilk: Take two slices of bread. Insert filling of your choice. Repeat. There—you've just made lunch for yourself *and* your wife. Better yet, accompany her to the doctor's office, then take her out for a bite to eat afterward.

READY TO RADIATE

When your wife reaches the radiation phase, she will most likely be in the home stretch of what breast cancer husband Bruce Bather calls the "triathlon of treatments." (Some women do get radiation in between rounds of chemo, or concurrent with chemo if Adriamycin is not in the mix.) Regardless of when the radiation takes place, your wife should lay the groundwork early on. Her surgeon should be able to recommend a radiation oncologist who frequently treats breast cancer patients, and she should visit this specialist in the first few weeks after diagnosis, when she is assembling her team of docs. Why do this before surgery and chemo? Because those two treatments could wipe out vital information about the patient's tumor that the radiation oncologist needs to obtain.

How does your wife know if she needs radiation in the first place? If she's having a lumpectomy, then she puts herself at great risk of a local recurrence if she does not have radiation. In fact, radiation will cut her odds of recurrence by 66 to 75 percent—a tremendous advantage. One surgeon told me of a woman whose (supremely selfish) husband did not want her to have radiation following her lumpectomy. He wanted her to become pregnant right away. She skipped radiation and conceived and bore a child. And sure enough, she had a recurrence of the cancer a couple of years later and had to have a mastectomy.

In addition, some mastectomy patients are candidates for radiation. A radiation oncologist might recommend treatment if the tumor is larger than 5 centimeters, if there are four or more positive lymph nodes, or if there were positive margins—that is, traces of cancer cells in the chest muscle after the mastectomy. The doctor might also suggest radiation for a premenopausal woman with lymph node involvement, for a woman with a small tumor but a lot of cancer cells in the lymphatic system or in the blood vessels, or for a woman with multiple cancers in one breast. In all these cases, radiation provides the same reduction in the risk of local recurrence.

So now you know why your wife might need radiation. But you (and she) may not know exactly what this treatment entails, and how it differs from chemotherapy. I know I didn't.

Don't worry, you'll find out soon enough. Chemotherapy consists of powerful drugs that seek to wipe out any trace of breast cancer cells throughout the body. Because chemotherapy treats the entire system, it's known as systemic treatment. Radiation refers to x-rays that stun cancer cells in the breast, chest wall, or armpit that may have escaped the surgeon's scalpel because they were too small to detect. That makes it local treatment, affecting only the part of the body that is radiated.

Like chemo, radiation goes on and on: 5 days of zapping a week, for 5 to 7 weeks. There's an initial consultation that lasts about an hour. Then there's the "simulation"—another hour or so devoted to pinpointing the exact target of radiation therapy. The radiation oncologist calculates the appropriate dosage and maps out the area of the chest and armpit that will get the zap. Marsha remembers how painstaking the effort was to determine exactly where the radiation should hit. Unless your wife strenuously objects, a technician will tattoo permanent blue dots—each about the size of a pinhead—

to designate the area in question; that way, treatment fields can be precisely set up each day. The goal is to hit the cancer cells dead-on and spare the normal cells as much as possible.

Then come the daily treatments, 2 minutes or so of anticancer radiation.

SETTING UP THE SCHEDULE

"I remember one guy so distinctly," Dr. Gage told me. "He came in, and as his wife was getting arranged, the first shot out of the hat was, 'So, what do you think? Six weeks and the whole thing is over, right? Could we start, like Tuesday? Tuesday would be good. And then 6 weeks from then

---

LAST ZAPS

Radiation was such a different treatment for us. After all sorts of chemo side effects, the doctors warned Marsha to gear up for the worst. Amazingly, she had practically no side effects. The days and weeks slipped by, and suddenly, it was time for the last set of radiation treatments, known as a boost—an extra dose for good measure, so to speak, delivered via machine or implants to the area where the breast cancer had been.

Is the boost really necessary? A couple of years ago, Europeans opened a large-scale trial, randomly assigning women to have a boost or no boost. The motivation wasn't exactly altruistic. It was a desire to reduce the amount of money spent on the extra dosages. "Because, you know, that's their tax dollars at work," observes Marsha's radiation oncologist Irene Gage, M.D., who practices at Sibley Memorial Hospital in Washington, D.C. "They actually proved very nicely that the boost helps."

On the last day of radiation, some centers hand out a diploma certifying the completion of the treatment, as if the woman had just graduated from high school. The center may have a little fête for the patient, too—a bell to ring, candy, or cupcakes to mark the milestone.

Some men may think their wives have graduated, too. Treatment is over, back to normal.

Not so fast, pal. See the chapter, The New Normal, on page 272.

would be, let me look at my calendar . . . '" And he's already got out his date book.

Dr. Gage looked at him and said, "Whoa, it's never going to be over. You can count on that, okay. Because even when it's over, it's not over."

She was talking about breast cancer, not radiation specifically. Thankfully, when radiation is over, it's over.

And it's not up to the husband to run the radiation schedule. Your wife, as always, is the boss. "I invite the patient to schedule it," says Dr. Gage. "I try to minimize the trauma. We do try to be accommodating. Why create stress about the time of the appointment?" Some women want to go in early before they head to their jobs. Some prefer midday appointments. Others like to stop by before driving afternoon carpools or on their way home from work.

In remote parts of the country, a woman may face a long drive every weekday for radiation, or may need to relocate to another town for the duration of her treatment. Since lumpectomy is always paired with radiation, a patient who has the choice of lumpectomy or mastectomy must cope with the inconvenience if she wants to preserve her breast. Without radiation, 4 out of 10 lumpectomy patients would experience a recurrence of cancer in the breast. Researchers in Canada have been trying to see if fewer doses of radiation do the trick, but results so far are inconclusive.

Is your wife (or are you) feeling impatient? A 7-day-a-week schedule is not advisable to speed things along. That's because normal breast tissue repairs itself during the weekend off. (Cancer cells don't fix themselves as efficiently.) On the flip side, taking a week off from radiation would be a bad idea, because over that stretch of time, the cancer cells could gather strength. And that would defeat the very purpose of radiation treatment.

WHAT'S IT LIKE?

In my support group, the advent of radiation prompted the same question that came up at the start of chemo: "What's it like?" (Which is a polite way of asking, "How bad is it?") I was the veteran in the group—my wife had already completed her radiation therapy. I could relate to their nervousness: I remember all too well that awful period of uncertainty before a new treatment. And having watched my wife go through the Big Three, I know the answer is the same for all breast cancer treatments: "It depends."

But I can clear up a few misconceptions about radiation. It does not make a patient radioactive (unless a radiation implant is used to treat only part of the breast with a concentrated dose; in that case, your wife would be hospitalized for a couple of days while the implant is active). Husbands (and wives) may also mistakenly think that radiation to the breast makes a patient nauseated or makes her lose her hair. Usually, the only hair that disappears would be on the breast itself, which makes radiation perhaps the only cancer treatment that provides a cosmetic benefit.

Radiation has far fewer side effects than decades ago, when the lungs or heart would have received an ample portion of the x-rays. But it's not a free ride. For some patients, radiation causes fatigue, the gradual onset of swelling and of shooting pains or discomfort in the breast, as well as itching, pinkness, burning, and sometimes peeling of the skin. (I go into more detail in the next section.) Your wife may have a slightly increased risk of breaking a rib were she to fall or have a violent cough after radiation treatment, but the break would heal normally. And a little scar tissue can occur in the lung right under the treated breast, just as pneumonia can leave a trace of scar tissue.

If the radiation is directed to the lymph nodes under the arm and at the base of the neck, it can slightly increase the risk of lymphedema, the swelling of the arm and hand that affects some breast cancer patients who've had lymph nodes removed.

Studies have not conclusively shown any increased risk of cancer in the other breast because of radiation. In extremely rare instances, Dr. Weiss notes, radiation can cause another type of cancer, but she hasn't seen this occur in the 15 years she has been in practice.

PICNIC OR PAIN?

Of the Big Three—surgery, chemo, and radiation—the zap is typically the weakest sister, especially compared with chemo. In fact, your wife's hair should start making its triumphant return during the days of radiation. Radiation also does not have quite the trauma associated with anesthesia and

GUY TALK

"Radiation just knocked Barbara out."

—RODNEY DORAND, 57
Pike Road, Alabama, describing his wife's reaction

surgery. Lots of women have told me that radiation was "a picnic" compared with the other treatments. Now I don't know about you, but I think of a picnic as a joyous celebration of food and nature on a sun-kissed meadow—not a visit to a doctor's office for an x-ray assault. The point is that many women don't come away from their daily dose feeling worse than when they went in, and in breast cancer world, that's a picnic.

Unfortunately, not every patient breezes through radiation. Dr. Gage believes that about half of her patients begin to feel better during radiation, even if they're still coping with side effects of just-completed chemotherapy. But the other half suffer extreme fatigue as the treatment continues. "I usually tell people I have no idea how they'll do," Dr. Gage says. "We'll find out together." That way, they don't count on feeling good—and aren't disappointed if they suffer side effects.

The tiredness associated with radiation is a bit mysterious. Could this really be fatigue that's left over from chemo? That may be true in some cases, but women who have not had chemo still report feeling tired during radiation treatment. Perhaps the therapy does indeed trigger a sense of weariness. The fatigue might also be a residue of the great stress your wife has suffered from all her treatments catching up with her in this last round of therapy. The daily disruption of her way-too-busy life for radiation appointments could contribute.

But it doesn't really matter what is making your wife tired. The point is that the fatigue is real and you should not think for a second that it's in your wife's head.

Actually, words like "fatigue" and "tired" may not do justice to what she's feeling. One patient told Dr. Gage: "Don't call it fatigue. Call it loss of initiative." Your wife may feel she's lost her zip, her get-up-and-go, her interest in life. Going to bed early or taking a nap doesn't always help.

In addition to fatigue, your wife may develop a burn and chafing in the radiated area. The doctor will recommend over-the-counter ointments and prescription creams that help; applying them from the beginning can make a huge difference. Marsha had what we affectionately called a "tit tan," but no real discomfort. Other women suffer. "I wasn't prepared for the burn," says Lawanna Robinson, 63. "Oh my, I was like a burn patient toward the end." She relied on Neosporin and an electric fan to keep her breast cool and comfortable. Another woman told me how her husband lovingly massaged her red, irritated skin with soothing salves.

Radiation might also make your wife's breast feel heavy. When she rolls over in bed, her breast may land on the mattress with a soft thump or an "ouch," making it difficult to drift off or jostling her from a sound sleep.

If you're not going to the treatments, you may be less inclined to sympathize. Don't make that mistake. And remember what I said about flowers all those chapters ago? It still holds true!

TIPS ➢ ➢ ➢

1. No, you don't have to go to every one of the 30-some radiation treatments, but it would be nice to show your face and meet the doc.
2. Urge your wife to schedule radiation to fit into her routine.
3. If your wife's breast is chafed and tender from radiation, put on some sexy music and rub in the soothing creams that the doctor recommends.

➢ BONUS TIP

A headset and some of your wife's favorite music will help pass the time as she awaits her daily dose.

Mysteries of Metastatic Disease

Living with uncertainty—and with hope

When football player Chris Spielman learned that his 30-year-old wife, Stefanie, had breast cancer, he says he felt as if Mark McGwire had slammed him in the head with a baseball bat.

(In case you're wondering, I did ask the 6-foot-tall, 230-pound Spielman why he went for a baseball image instead of one from football. He said he was trying to imagine the world's most powerful knockout punch.)

A couple of years later, doctors told Stefanie that her breast cancer had recurred—as metastatic disease. The cancer cells that had begun multiplying in her breast had spread to her lungs.

This time, Chris felt as if he'd been hit by something far mightier than McGwire's Louisville Slugger. But he figured that he could be strong; he could fight like he fought before. The day after the diagnosis, he went to drop his daughter off at school in the morning. Driving home, he suddenly didn't feel much like a fighter anymore. A wave of worry and pain and fear swept over him. He had to pull the car to the curb. "I couldn't move," he remembers. He curled up into a fetal ball. "I threw up the white flag," he says. "I gave myself a little bit too much credit on how much strength I had to handle this situation. I looked to God and said, 'I can't do this. You win. It's in Your control. Give me the strength to do what You want me to do.'" Within an hour, he was back in attack mode, but with a new battle plan: "I knew I wasn't the source of my strength. God was the source of strength."

No matter what a breast cancer husband's religious beliefs, if his wife has been diagnosed with metastatic disease, he can surely identify with Chris Spielman. The news is shattering, and it will take all of your strength—and then some—to cope.

HOW DID THIS HAPPEN?

Metastatic disease means that the cancer that began in the breast has spread or "metastasized," typically hitching a ride in the bloodstream or lymphatic system and then finding a hospitable home elsewhere in the body. Unfortunately, there's still a great deal that doctors don't know about the journey of cancer cells, and why they do or don't thrive in a new locale. Perhaps they lay dormant for a long spell until conditions become ripe for them to begin growing again. But one thing doctors do know: Breast cancer cells are far more insidious once they take up residence in a distant site. Many women live for years with metastatic disease. Others are not as fortunate.

Between 2 and 5 percent of women are found to have metastatic disease when they are first diagnosed with breast cancer—between 4,000 and 10,000 of the 200,000 or so annually diagnosed cases. That's what all those initial scans are for—looking at your wife's bones and liver and lungs and the like for signs of cancer. But the vast majority of times, metastatic breast cancer is found many months (or even years) after the initial diagnosis, most likely after a woman has visited the doctor complaining of such symptoms as bone pain or shortness of breath or a cough she can't shake.

Doctors do yearly mammography and regular exams to monitor for signs of recurrence; that's what the guidelines are at this time. Some docs do blood work as well to check for abnormalities. A decade or so ago, doctors performed annual bone and CAT scans, too, but the scans almost always turned up something—and the spots and other findings usually proved to be benign. So cancer doctors don't extensively test for metastatic disease unless there are symptoms, because the truth is that, at this time, there is virtually no hope for a cure,

(continued on page 250)

RANDY'S RULES

If you're looking for instruction in the art of living with metastatic disease, I don't think you could do any better than to sit by Randy Harper's feet and listen a spell.

Randy and his wife, Hilary, live in Auburn Township, a semirural suburb of Cleveland. He's originally from Clarksville, "a little bitty town in Georgia." Hilary's from Cleveland. Randy is 44; Hilary is 40. They're the parents of two: a son, 14, and a daughter, 9. Randy is a musician who produces ad jingles. Before her cancer, Hilary had worked as a sales rep for a telecommunications firm, and Randy boasts that she was one of the company's star sellers.

Hilary's cancer diagnosis in September 2000 "was kinda wild," Randy remembers. She had a grade III invasive tumor. "Anything that could be bad about this cotton-pickin' tumor, it was bad," he says. But the tumor, as it turned out, wasn't the worst of the news. Hilary was hoping to take part in a clinical trial that would include a bone marrow transplant, so she had to have her bone marrow tested to qualify. The marrow came back positive. Cancer was in her bones. When the doctors did their first set of scans, a spot turned up on her lungs. It was negative. Then a couple of years later, doctors did more scans and, as Randy remembers, "That lung spot lit up like a lightbulb. Turns out it was malignant."

Now their life is a succession of clinical trial chemos and doctor's visits. "The side effects of this chemo she's on right now are not that bad," Randy says. The results weren't that bad, either. The tumor that was found in her lungs last year had begun to shrink. When I recently got back in touch with Randy, doctors had found two brain lesions, but they appeared to be responding to treatment. "Our last scans were encouraging," Randy said, although the oncologist was still concerned. Through it all, Randy has learned to be wary of predictions. At the very beginning, he looked up the survival statistics for Hilary's type of tumor, and he found "up to 5 years' survival."

"I was not a very happy camper," he says. "You know, it pissed me off." A lump formed in his throat.

"If you want to know exactly what I said," Randy recalls, "I said, this is bullshit." And it was, in a way. As he dug deeper, he found that the statistics were over 10 years old, and that advances in treatment had been made.

At the time, he told Hilary that he was afraid. "You know what I was afraid of, honest to God, and what I'm afraid of more than anything else? I'm afraid of leaving stones unturned."

Since then, he's relaxed a bit. "I'm not as tense about that kind of stuff. Plus, we have good doctors. I know they're pretty straight shooters."

So the Harpers live their suburban life, with kids and chemo and a heavier burden of chores on Randy. "I'm pretty decent at throwing in the wash, but I'm useless when it comes to folding it," he laments. "If she gives me the real, real dirty look, I know it's my turn to go." And her turn to fold.

His son, Corey, has asked, "Will we lose Mom?"

Randy says, "There's that possibility. But there's also the possibility that we won't lose her to this. There's also the possibility she steps in front of a bus. We can't play that game."

I ask him how hard it is to be the support for his wife in her fight with metastatic disease.

"My job is so easy," Randy answers. "I don't have the hard job. She's got the tough job.

"Can it be beat? I don't know yet. They tell us we can't be cured because we're metastatic. I'm not giving up and I don't think Hilary is either." First, because he wants to hold on to hope. And second, because he fears that giving up would open the door for bitterness to creep in. "I never lived that way, and I don't intend to start now. You have to look at it like a chronic disease. If I looked at it any other way, I would be cheating Hilary.

"Now I look in the mirror once in a while and say to myself, 'What if?' And that does scare the heck out of me. It scares me because I don't even remember my life without her."

"Do you dwell on that?" I ask.

"God, no. There's too much work to do, she's got too much to do; there's so much that both of us have to live for and live with on a daily basis that keeps us up and keeps us going."

So the Harpers cope with a range of emotions, aided by hearty doses of Randy's southern-fried humor. Sometimes, Randy says, people have hinted that he doesn't take this cancer thing seriously enough. How can he be cracking jokes and playing music with his buddies in a bar every so often and exuding cockeyed optimism?

"My response would be," says Randy, "how in the heck would you expect me to be any other way?"

just symptom management. As Washington, D.C., breast surgeon Cynthia Drogula, M.D., puts it, "The treatment for metastatic disease is symptomatic, so why know about it before symptoms appear? Why not be dumb and happy? Patients hate to hear that. Early detection has been drummed into them. And when they find out you're not going to be CAT scanning them every year looking for recurrences, they can't believe it. But sadly, it doesn't make a difference. So finding out before you have symptoms really doesn't help."

You won't hear a whole lot about metastatic disease in the world of breast cancer activists. "We used to have the 'C' word," says Memorial Sloan-Kettering social worker Roz Kleban, talking about the days when fear and ignorance kept people from even saying the name of the disease. "Now we have the 'M' word. Thank God, the bulk of all breast cancers do not metastasize; the bulk of all patients go on to live long, healthy lives." These survivors are often at the head of breast cancer organizations, and they're terrified of the notion of stage IV disease, Kleban says. The Young Survival Coalition, based in New York City, is one exception—a breast cancer group that doesn't shy away from tackling metastatic disease in its meetings and workshops.

Even the medical community seems a little skittish about the "M" word. When breast cancer survivors go to doctors with symptoms that could be the result of metastatic disease, the docs sometimes look for other causes, perhaps because they don't want to face the devastating news that their patient has had a recurrence. A couple of years after her breast cancer diagnosis, Lynn Grogan developed back pains following a ranch vacation. Perhaps riding a horse all day was the culprit, the physician first postulated. The doctor was wrong. Lynn Grogan's breast cancer had metastasized to her bones. But the instinct to avoid a cancer diagnosis is understandable. "It's not quite as emotionally trying for me to give bad news as it is for a patient to receive it, but it's pretty damn close," says Mikkael Sekeres, M.D., co-editor of the book *Facing Cancer* and an assistant professor in the hematology-oncology department at the Cleveland Clinic Lerner College of Medicine. "I want to avoid having to do that as much as possible."

But if that is the news, you don't want a doctor who sugarcoats. Oncologist Carolyn Hendricks, M.D., who treats breast cancer patients in Montgomery County, Maryland, delivers what she calls "a tough but necessary" message to a patient newly diagnosed with metastatic disease: "Make a short list of what's important to you, and don't spend a minute with someone who's not important or with things that aren't important. Stressed at work? Table it. Family issues? Deal with them or let them go. Whether you can live 10 months or 10 years, don't spend time with things that diminish the quality of your life."

WHAT TO HOPE FOR

Vickie Girard, 50, a petite former secretary for General Motors, got her virtual death sentence in 1992. Doctors told her that the cancer they had found in her breast 3 years earlier had spread to her head, neck, shoulder, spine, breastbone, and first rib. Her oncologist gave her maybe a year to live if she had her ovaries removed and tried hormonal therapy. Chemotherapy was not recommended. The doctor told her that chemo "would destroy the quality of whatever quantity of life" she had left.

When Vickie described her diagnosis to me, more than a decade had passed from the time she learned that her cancer had metastasized. Back in the gloom of 1992, she vowed that if even 1 in 100 women in her situation could survive, then she was going to be in that exclusive club. So she went out and found a different set of docs, who treated her with chemo, "nutritional support," and mind-body therapies. "We are each individuals," she stresses in her inspirational speeches. "We are not a set of statistics." Besides, she notes with a grin, "if God wanted us to know how long we have to live, He would have sent us to this earth with an expiration date."

Nonetheless, there are statistics in books and on the Internet, and you will undoubtedly come across them. You will most likely read that the average survival time after a diagnosis of metastatic disease is 2 to 3 years. Some women die within a year of diagnosis. About one in three patients will live for 5 years. One in 10 women survive a decade or more. You will also learn that metastatic disease in the bones is considered less threatening than in organs like the lungs or liver, which aren't called "vital" for nothing. Their role in breathing and manufacturing blood, for example, can be compromised by the spread of cancer cells. You'll learn that a woman who has metastatic disease at the first diagnosis, or who has a recurrence shortly after treatment ends for

GUY TALK

"Ninety-nine percent of the time the best thing to do is just give her a hug. As far as saying, 'Don't worry, it'll be okay'—well, you don't know, she doesn't know, and that could make her more upset."

—BOB HEIL, 39
Wausau, Wisconsin, whose wife, Brenda, was found to have metastatic disease 14 years after her initial breast cancer diagnosis

local breast cancer, faces a bleaker future than a woman who has gone years from the end of treatment before being diagnosed with metastatic disease.

But the numbers you find, even those on the most up-to-date Web sites, reflect the past, not the present, and certainly not the future. "All the statistics don't take into account what is going to be," explains Roz Kleban, who runs support groups for women with metastatic disease. "I warn patients, don't go on the Internet indiscriminately. You hang in there with advanced disease until the next thing comes along. You need to hang in there and as much as possible, stay within the now."

"If you look at the statistical curve," says Don Shields, whose wife, Carol, battled metastatic breast cancer, "there is a tail that goes way out to the right. It says that a few people are going to live quite long. Those tails are quite significant to the individual." Three times, doctors told his wife that she had only 6 months to live. Hearing those words "caused us considerable grief, as you may imagine," Don says. "But always something has come along to take away that prognosis—a new treatment, perhaps, that has improved Carol's quality of life and extended it."

Doctors who treat cancer agree. "It's not a false hope" to want to be at the end of the long tail of the survival curve, says Dr. Sekeres. And indeed, the outcome of an individual patient's case may defy all expectations.

There are women with metastatic disease who receive treatment that puts their cancer in remission, and they live out their lives "free of disease." "Free of disease means there is no evidence of disease on exam or by x-rays that we can determine," explains Bruce Haffty, M.D., a radiation oncologist at Yale University. The cancer cells may still be present but aren't numerous enough to be detected. If a patient with metastatic disease lives many years and eventually dies of another cause—does that mean she has been cured? At the very least, she wasn't a victim of breast cancer.

But in the back of your mind, you must realize that if Vickie Girard was the lucky 1 out of 100 who defied her prognosis, the other unlucky 99 women also wanted to beat the odds.

PICK A TREATMENT

Rob Sawyer was stunned when he and his girlfriend first met with the oncologist to discuss the cancer that had been found in her breast, her lymph nodes, her liver, and her bones.

"I'm an engineer," says Sawyer, 34, who lives in Haverhill, Massachusetts. "Engineers see things in black and white. You have a problem, you try to solve it." He expected his girlfriend's doctor to say, "You are a 40-year-old woman. You have metastatic disease. Here's the best treatment." Instead, her oncologist was popping up Web pages, looking at drugs in trial, and admitting that she didn't know whether a particular treatment would work or not. "I'm not happy about it," Sawyer says. But he's made his peace with uncertainty.

Clearly, your wife (or girlfriend) does need an oncologist who has treated a lot of metastatic disease and who is familiar with cutting-edge therapies. Depending on where the metastasis has occurred, radiation or chemotherapy may be in order. Surgery is sometimes recommended. "I had a craniotomy—they opened up my head and took the cancer out surgically," says Tracy Hill, 36, who was diagnosed 4 years ago, of her recent brain lesion. "Amazing what you'll put up with when you want to live, ain't it?"

Then there are hormonal treatments like tamoxifen, and other experimental procedures. You may latch on to a study you read about in the local paper or hear about one on the evening news. "There's new stuff out every day," says oncologist Adam Brufsky, M.D., who codirects the Magee-Womens Hospital Breast Cancer Program in Pittsburgh. But many of the studies describe tests on animals, not human beings. Translating from animal to human can take 5, 6, 7 years. Even then the treatment may not work for cancer patients.

But it never hurts to ask.

LIFE STILL GOES ON

Even with metastatic disease. Your wife may tire more easily. She may be in a degree of pain, from moderate to massive. But I interviewed couples who are—well, optimistic is not quite the right word. But maybe "realistic" is. They're hopeful of having many years together. They're hopeful that new treatments will be developed that would be beneficial. But they are also facing a very different reality than couples where the wife has local breast cancer. In that instance, you're talking about perhaps 8 or 10 months of treatment. With metastatic disease, there may be years of treatments. "Women need to look at it as a chronic disease that warrants continuous monitoring," says nurse Lillie Shockney.

Your wife may not be able to do as much in the household as she did before. She will need your support. "Have I seen men rise to that occasion?" Roz Kleban says. "Absolutely. I see magnificent partners go through this thing hand in hand, talking about *our* treatment, *our* appointments, *our* tests."

She pauses for a minute, then adds, "but it's tremendously difficult."

Your wife may be overwhelmed with worry; she may be self-absorbed because that's what happens when you're fighting an illness like metastatic breast cancer. Or she may conceal her true condition from you, not sharing the degree of her pain and suffering, because she doesn't want to frighten you. Again, your job is not to be the cheerleader but to try to give her hope if you can. You can remind her of any positive comments the doctor might have said about the efficacy of her treatments. But you have no right to expect her to be positive all the time. "A negative attitude is not good and not bad," says Kleban. "It's just normal." When people might marvel at how good she looks, your wife shouldn't feel she has to live up to anyone's expectations. She can say, "I feel like crap."

And when people tell her to buck up, she doesn't have to oblige with a show of optimism. She can say, "You can walk in my shoes and tell me whether you'd have a positive attitude." You can say the same thing if your friends are making you feel as if you don't have the right to feel bad.

Your wife may joke sardonically about the woman you'll marry when she's gone, making barbed comments like, "We just got a new kitchen floor, and I'll be goddamned if the second Mrs. Jones is going to walk on my floor." Social worker Roz Kleban has heard women talk about such things and laugh. But she doesn't suggest that husbands join in. "I've never heard men make those jokes," she says. If you feel the need to engage in a little dark humor for stress relief, that's understandable. But try to do so with your male buddies, Kleban says, not with your wife.

If you and your wife have kids, you may be the one who talks to them about what's going on. If the doctors haven't given up hope, you shouldn't either. Say that Mom has a serious disease, that the doctors have lots of medicines to treat it, and that they're going to take good care of her. That's all true. If your child asks whether Mommy is going to die, you can say, "Not now, and we hope not for many years. The doctors will let us know if they can't do anything more to help Mom." That reassures a child that Mom won't suddenly be gone—and that if things look worse, you will tell them.

Encourage your wife to try any of the complementary therapies she might have tried before—yoga, meditation, guided imagery, healing touch. Just as important, you might want to follow the example of a husband who shared his philosophy at a recent breast cancer seminar. He tells his wife, who has metastatic disease, to do two things every day: "Do something just for you. I don't need to know what it is. It doesn't have to be with anybody. And find something that makes you laugh your fanny off."

It may help you and your wife to have a role model—someone like Vickie Girard, who confounded the experts; you can read her story in her book, *No Place Like Hope*. Or Lance Armstrong, who was diagnosed in 1996 with an aggressive form of testicular cancer that had spread to his abdomen, lungs, and brain. After 3 months of treatment, he went on to win the Tour de France again and again. And don't be discouraged by setbacks. Vickie Girard's cancer recently recurred and she is taking chemotherapy again. But she remains upbeat: "This is not the end of the road, but a bump in the road."

It may also help if you and your wife can find time for physical affection. "Don't leave sex in the closet," advises Kleban. The Spielmans didn't. Stefanie Spielman actually got pregnant after her diagnosis with metastatic disease and gave birth to a healthy baby. "You'll have to ask her about sex," her husband, Chris, says sheepishly. "It might be better. I don't know. I can't remember what it was like before breast cancer." (But any breast cancer patient, regardless of the stage of her disease, should ask her doctors about the risks of pregnancy and its rush of estrogen.)

Through it all, the breast cancer husband still has to find time for himself. You may feel guilty doing things you enjoy, because you are not the one battling metastatic disease. But how can you not take a little time for yourself?

"I'm living more for myself, and it makes both of us feel better," says Jeff Hill, 36, Tracy's husband. She had been diagnosed with breast cancer in 2000, then had a metastatic recurrence a year later. When I spoke to Jeff, Tracy was getting once-a-week chemo that knocks her down for a couple of days, but "she deals with it pretty well, probably better than I would," Jeff says.

"Seeing her tired and sick just drove me nuts," he adds. He tried to live as if things were normal, and his wife would accuse him of "trying to pretend we're normal people."

"Maybe that's what I was trying to do," Jeff says. "But it didn't work." Because he couldn't escape the reach of cancer, he was angry and miserable. "I like to fix things," he says. "I build race cars for a living. But I can't fix her." (Now there's a familiar refrain.) "And that really pissed me off. I want answers. These doctors all say, 'We don't know.'"

He's been so mad that he's wanted to punch walls—"which is so unlike me. It's a blur. The last 3 years have just been nonstop cancer. I was just this lump."

Then Jeff went on a scuba diving trip—he's an avid diver—and a guy he met told him, "Get your ass in gear—she's not dead, you're not dead. Go have some fun." Jeff took those words to heart. Now he and Tracy are thinking of selling their Westwood, New Jersey, home and moving to the shore. "Life's too short," says Jeff. "You have to live life while you can."

TIPS ➢ ➢ ➢

1. At a local breast cancer center, ask about support groups for women with metastatic disease.
2. Ask your insurer to assign a case manager to handle all the queries about your wife's bills. Having a point person who knows the details can be helpful.
3. Caregivers—that would be you—need a respite from metastatic disease. "There are no extra points given to men in heaven for doing it all," says nurse Lillie Shockney. Ask for help, and even time off, when you need it.

➢ BONUS TIP

Don't be scared by statistics you find on the Web about the predicted life span for breast cancer patients with metastatic disease. The numbers are based on past treatments, not current (or soon-to-be-available) therapies.

Facing Death

Holding on, letting go

On a chilly evening in May, 1,365 women and 112 men were finishing up dinner and thinking about how much fun it would (or wouldn't) be to spend the night in sleeping bags in a tent city. On a field of brambles. With a huge power generator emitting a steady hum.

This was the scene at the Avon Walk for Breast Cancer in Boston.

I was one of the small contingent of guys, walking to pay tribute to my wife's courage, to raise money for education, treatment, patient support, and research, and to meet some of the other fellows giving up their weekend to trudge 26.2 miles or more (for those who fear no blisters, there's a 39.3-mile option).

Dave Quemere was one of the men I met. He was 46 but looked younger, with an open and friendly face, reddish hair, a mustache, a nice grin. We chatted after dinner, as the sun set and the sky turned purple and red and then inky black.

I asked him to tell me his story. And his story turned out to be the story that no breast cancer husband wants to hear.

Dave's wife, Donna, was diagnosed with breast cancer 11 years ago, when she was 39, the mother of a newborn and a 3-year-old. Doctors found a 4-centimeter tumor and lymph node involvement. She was treated with a mastectomy, chemo, and radiation, and all appeared to be well. For 2½ years she was in remission.

Then Donna found herself growing short of breath. She knew her body, and she knew something was wrong. The cancer had returned—in her lungs. She did some more chemo, and that gave her a few months of seemingly good health. But the cancer again showed up in her lungs and was found in her liver, too. She tried a bone marrow transplant. "She was sick as a dog," Dave remembers. She had 3 really good months after the procedure, but the whole time she wondered, "When is it coming back?"

Her cancer reappeared in August 1997. Donna added her name to a lottery waiting list for a new experimental drug. For months she waited. When she finally "won" the lottery, her oncologist told her that she had only 2 weeks to live, and that the drug would take a month to have any effect. And that it would make her sick to her stomach. "Either you can do that," her doctor said, "or you can be with the kids and enjoy the time left." Donna said, "That's it. I want to be with my kids."

She decided what to do on her own, Dave says, and told him her decision, adding, "I hope you agree." He said, "How can I disagree? I know what the doctor said."

Some members of her family weren't as understanding. They wanted to know why she was giving up. Dave didn't see it that way at all. "I told her, 'Donna, this is the bravest decision you ever made.'"

In terrible pain, she refused pain medication as long as she could, lest the drugs muddy her mind. Finally, she relented; a hospice nurse gave her what is called "breakthrough medication," Dave recalls. The idea behind this treatment is that if the pain from the cancer has raced far ahead, a breakthrough drug like liquid morphine could catch up with the pain and vanquish it.

Some people recover from the stress of such drugs. "She was too far gone," Dave says bitterly. He is a believer in hospice care—in fact, he is a social worker for a hospice—but he thinks the nurse should have explained that the drug could knock his wife into an unconscious state from which she might never emerge. He wishes he had known so that he and Donna could have had one last conversation, and he hopes that any husband in his position understands the implications of a breakthrough drug.

"I felt so cheated," Dave says. "She never woke up, except to say a few words." And then she was gone. She had set two final goals: to live long enough to see her younger son's fifth birthday, and then to see him start kindergarten. Conor turned 5 on March 10, 1998; she planned and attended his party. He would start school in the fall. She died on April 9.

Dave wiped a few tears from his eyes as we talked. Then, his emotions took hold. He broke down sobbing and said in a voice so low I could barely make out the words: "I hate this fucking disease."

His words stung like an icy wind. They are a harsh rejoinder to the upbeat breast cancer message that groups like Avon promote: that with early detection, women can beat this disease, and that survivors feel their life after breast cancer is richer or more rewarding than it was before. Those statements are certainly true. Yet that is only part of the truth about breast cancer. Each year, some 40,000 women die of the disease. I'm sure if you could ask them, they would agree with Dave 100 percent.

DIFFICULT DECISIONS

How do you cope when you fear that the end is near?

You do the same thing you did when you and your wife had hope for a disease-free future. You talk to each other, you share your views, you seek the help of a therapist if denial is getting in the way (which is easier said than done, especially for a man who feels he has failed to protect his wife from the ravages of breast cancer). Above all, you respect your wife's right to make the decisions that are right for her.

That's what I learned when I spoke to the gifted novelist Carol Shields and her husband, Don, last year. A Pulitzer Prize winner for her book *The Stone Diaries*, Carol had been diagnosed with stage III breast cancer in 1998. "Just before Christmas," her husband recalls. "It was not a good thing." The lesion itself was quite far along, and all of the 19 lymph nodes taken tested positive for cancer. One doctor told Carol that she had less than a year to live if she did not take chemotherapy, and perhaps 2 or 3 years if she did opt for the treatment. "That didn't seem like very much," Carol said. Experimental treatments might prolong her life, but could make her remaining days miserable.

The book *How We Die* by Sherwin Nuland, M.D., became the couple's bible. The clinical professor at Yale University states emphatically that the patient should be the one to make decisions about treatment. "He or she should not feel obligated to the people they love to go into these treatments or prolong their lives and their own discomfort and distress," Don says. "We're trying to follow his recommendations to the best of our ability. Sometimes it's not the easiest thing, you know." That's putting it mildly.

"I definitely have had some treatments that I wouldn't have had if Don hadn't wanted them so badly," said Carol. "But that seems like a fair tradeoff."

Three times the doctors told her she had 3 to 6 months to live. The first two times, she elected to try a new treatment, and the treatment gave her a temporary reprieve. In one instance, the breast cancer had shown up in her liver. Doctors were able to cut off the blood supply to the tumor and then inject poison into it. Carol was in agony and distress. After 7 weeks or so, Don says, "my family was very concerned that we'd made the wrong decision. We were prepared to say we'd made a mistake." Then Carol woke up one morning and felt okay. And her liver was functioning.

But metastatic breast cancer can be a brutal beast. The disease again began interfering with Carol's liver function; she elected to try an experimental therapy that involved high doses of steroids. Her liver function went from abnormal to normal. But the steroids began to affect her ability to think; they altered her appearance, too, as steroids can do.

Carol could not stand to live with those side effects. "She elected to quit halfway through," Don said when I spoke to him early in 2003. "We respected that. She was the one being injured by the treatment."

On July 16, 2003, Carol Shields died of breast cancer. She was 67. After her death, Don sent me a note about facing life without her. "I am in France now for 3 weeks, at our home in Burgundy," he wrote. "Everywhere I look about this old house, I see Carol's presence. I am in a new phase of my cancer-induced relationship with Carol."

TRYING TO TALK

Holding on. Letting go. Those are the terrible twins of terminal breast cancer. Carol and Don were able to talk about the possibility of her death, and of the risks and benefits of experimental drugs. Not every couple can be that forthright. Patricia Spicer, an oncology social worker for the national organization CancerCare, has seen couples where the woman is dying and the husband or boyfriend knows it, but can't admit it. "You feel for the husband in these situa-

HOW AND WHEN TO TALK ABOUT HOSPICE

How does a breast cancer patient know when the time has come to stop hoping for remission or cure and to pursue a different kind of care?

For health insurers, the answer is simple. When a doctor believes that a patient has less than 6 months to live, Medicare deems the patient eligible for hospice care—end-of-life care that seeks to manage the patient's pain and other symptoms, and to provide psychological and spiritual support for the patient and family members. Many private insurers follow the same guidelines. In 2002, hospices served 885,000 terminally ill Americans. Half of them were cancer patients.

But how does your wife find the courage to raise the subject of hospice? And how do you find the strength to support her? Those are questions with no easy answers. She may be ready to face the inevitable, or she may be in denial. The husband, and the doctor, too, might be deniers. "Some physicians want to fight to the bitter end," says Karen Higgins of the Hospice Foundation of America. "They don't want to give up." If your wife has advanced breast cancer, perhaps she might want to ask her oncologist early on—tell me if and when you think the time has come to consider hospice care. But this topic may be too painful for her to raise. "All the husband can do is support his wife's decision," Higgins emphasizes. "Ultimately, the wife and the oncologist have to make the decision," agrees social worker Dave Quemere, who works for a hospice and whose own wife sought hospice care at the end of her struggle with breast cancer. "The husband runs the risk of being scorned by the wife if he suggests that they have tried everything, and maybe it is time to look to hospice. My advice to the husband is to speak to the doctor about how well or poorly treatment is going. If the doctor feels hospice is needed, the doc can suggest it to the wife."

If your wife is ready to think about hospice, you will probably be the one

tions," says Spicer. "There is help available, and it is so hard for them to reach out and get it. It's that John Wayne syndrome—'I'm supposed to be the big, strong guy.'"

In other ways, he's like a little child, clinging to the power of magical

---

who does the research. The National Hospice and Palliative Care Organization has a database of local groups on its Web site: www.nhpco.org. Or you can call the group at (800) 658-8898. You may have several choices, or you may have but one. At all hospice groups, the goal is to provide home-based care if possible, and that is how 80 percent of hospice patients receive care. Depending on the hospice staff, regular visitors will include a doctor, a nurse, a social worker, a chaplain, and a health aide, as well as a volunteer to help with anything from running errands to organizing records. In addition, some hospices have a facility where patients can stay if home care is not possible. For more information about a particular hospice, you and your wife may want to speak to the family member of a past patient. Typically, that can be arranged.

Once hospice care begins, the medical team will work to control your wife's pain while keeping her lucid. "It can take a couple of days to find the perfect balance," says Jon Radulovic, a spokesman for the National Hospice and Palliative Care Organization. If a patient enters a hospice program only a day or two before death, as sometimes happens, it may be too late to achieve that goal—and certainly too late for the patient and her family to benefit from the full range of hospice services. Regardless of the timing, the husband might quietly ask about what happens when the patient dies. Each hospice has its own procedures—including a plan for disposing of your wife's supply of unused drugs.

Bob Marovich remembers how startled he was when a hospice staffer came to his house after his wife's death, swept up her chemo pills and other medications, and flushed them down the toilet. But aside from that unsettling scene, he was deeply grateful for hospice care: "We knew that if something was wrong, there was somebody on call to help at any time." That was a comfort to Bob and to his wife, Pat, in her dying days.

thinking. "Husbands think, 'If I don't talk about it, it won't happen,'" says Mary Hughes, a nurse at M.D. Anderson Cancer Center in Houston. The truth is that death has more power when you don't talk about it. It looms like an omnipotent spirit. But it may seem easier to cling to false hope than to face a bitter truth.

Bernie Smith, 67, of Annandale, Virginia, remembers all too well how hard it was to face the unfaceable. His wife, Jacqui, was diagnosed with cancer at age 41. She had a lumpectomy and radiation, and 7½ years of good health. But then, the disease came back; the cancer had metastasized to her lungs.

Jacqui feared that others would give up hope, and she wanted to hold on. So she deputized her husband as her "minister of optimism."

"You must never give up," Jacqui told him.

And there was a time of hopefulness. After chemotherapy treatments, the doctor said there were no new lesions. That was December 17, 1991. Her next appointment was set for April. She died on March 3.

"We tried never to give up hope," Bernie says. "Once she deputized me, I couldn't give up hope. I could never show any sign that we were going to lose." Even when Jacqui agreed to hospice care, Bernie was in denial. He'd talk to her about their next trip—to Scotland, it would be. But in his heart, he knew. In those final days, he told his darling Jacqui, "I'm a better person because of you." And she said, "Oh, I know that, and the children know that."

Bernie pauses. "Everyone knew it but me."

When Bernie told me his story, his wife had been gone for more than a decade. But she was still a presence in his life. He was sitting in the bedroom that Jacqui had decorated—interior design was her career and her passion. The retired Department of the Army civilian has gone on to found the Men's Crusade Against Breast Cancer, an organization that raises money to fight the disease that took his wife—"because if we were losing that many men in a war, we'd definitely spend more to keep them alive."

But when I heard the tears in his voice, I could tell he still feels that he fell short as a minister of optimism. "My mother said, 'You won't get over it,'" Bernie remembers. "'But you'll learn to live with it.'" She was right on both counts.

A DATE WITH ELEANOR ROOSEVELT

David Kupfer had a similar crisis—torn between optimism and pessimism. In fact, the Arlington, Virginia, psychologist had many crises in his 2 years as a breast cancer boyfriend. At age 36, his fiancée, Cathy Hainer, was diagnosed with stage IV breast cancer. The two of them explored every option for treatment together. Cathy chronicled her experiences in a series of deeply moving and darkly funny articles for *USA Today*, where she worked as a reporter.

"We were united in ignorance," says David, 51, who now counsels couples who are coping with breast cancer. "We knew we didn't know. We knew they didn't know. I was a research collaborator and I gave my opinions. But the decision was 100 percent hers."

A neighbor said that when his wife was diagnosed with breast cancer, "I just decided she wasn't going to die." And she didn't.

David wasn't quite that positive about the outcome of Cathy's disease. "Am I being negative because I'm not saying she won't die?" he asked himself. "Or am I just being realistic? Cathy was stage IV when she was diagnosed. The woman across the street wasn't.

"It requires an attitude that fits the reality," says David. "And you have to be okay when people around you say you are too optimistic or too pessimistic." Because really, what you want to be is realistic.

Yet he recognizes that in some ways he was too much of an optimist. "I made the mistake of thinking that knowledge can cure breast cancer," he says. David thought if he kept pushing for one more treatment, one more test, maybe that would make a difference.

After an initial round of chemotherapy, Cathy was found to have "no evidence of disease." But that hopeful phrase is not the same as "no disease." It means only that the doctors could not find any cancer cells. Months later, the cancer recurred in Cathy's brain and bones.

David could not accept the facts of the case, or the awful fact that nothing could be done. He wanted the doctors to do another scan so they'd know exactly where the metastatic cancer was. The doctors told him that really wouldn't help. It wouldn't help them know which medications to give Cathy to stop the pain, and it wouldn't stop the cancer from consuming her body. "It

GUY TALK

"I go to bed 2 or 3 hours after Carol. I find that a long and lonely time. Most days I go to bed with tears in my eyes."

—DON SHIELDS, 68
Vancouver, speaking of the final months of his wife's 4½-year battle with breast cancer

was hard for me to believe that they didn't want to know where, or to what degree, the cancer was spreading," David says. A month before her death, he was still pushing for more tests. A doctor took him aside and told him that more tests would not give them useful information.

Still, David kept fighting. "I would latch on to stupid things to make me feel like I was on top of things," he says. "For Cathy, it was the dosage of steroids. Her brain would swell, and the steroids would keep her brain from swelling. That was the thing I identified that was keeping her alive."

Each day, he would dash home from work. He would grill Cathy's father, who stayed with them, or the health aide on duty: When had she taken her pills? What was the dose? Were the pills cut up the right way?

When Cathy finally decided to ask for hospice care, the hospice nurse told the couple that the plan was to taper off the steroids. And that if fluid were to build up in her lungs, the hospice wouldn't rush her to the emergency room. Rather, its medical staff would assess the situation and decide on treatment to keep her comfortable.

"I felt guilty," David says. "I had been the fix-it man, making sure she had the right dose, powerful enough to keep her brain the right size—and to keep her alive forever.

"My tendency as a guy is to hold on. What I had to learn is the letting go part."

David remembers holding Cathy's hand when she passed away. "When she died, it was so peaceful," he says. They had had 2 frenetic, frantic years of running from doctor to doctor and searching for cures, from mainstream to magical. And finally, stripped of hope for a miraculous recovery, Cathy felt at peace. In a way that he couldn't have imagined, David was at peace, too. "The greatest gift I got from Cathy was that I did learn how to let go," he says. "I don't think of death as a bad thing anymore. I don't glorify it. But death was obviously a higher level of cure. And Cathy taught me to accept her death."

Indeed, Cathy was ready for her journey to the unknown. She drew up a list of all the dearly departed souls she was hoping to get together with. Her mom, who had died of breast cancer, was number one. Eleanor Roosevelt was high up as well. "We joked that Eleanor Roosevelt must have a huge staff, arranging meetings in the afterlife," David says.

But accepting the inevitability of death doesn't automatically bring tranquility and calm. "What am I supposed to do?" Cathy asked her fiancé at one point. "Wait to die?"

"Well, yes and no," David told her. "You can go for a walk, you can write another article, you can decide which friend you want to spend time with.

"No, you don't have to just wait. But yeah, you do have to wait."

A WOMAN IN DENIAL

The man is not always the one who has a hard time letting go. "Sandy refused to deal with any possibility that she would die," says Bob Miller of his wife. She had been diagnosed with breast cancer when she was 42. About 13 years later, she began complaining of hip and back pain. The doctors did test after test and found nothing—until the cancerous tumor in her hip grew big enough to be discovered.

Bob is a doctor in North Canton, Ohio; he works in critical care. "I see a lot of death and dying," he says. "I realize how fragile life is." He had always worried that the cancer would come back one day. And he wanted to make Sandy happy. "I took her all over the world, because that's what she wanted." They went to China, India, and France. To England, Italy, and Turkey. To Greece, Peru, and Costa Rica.

So he did not have regrets about the way they lived their life. But he has regrets about the way Sandy's life ended. "I think her mode was generally to deny," he says. "I bought a digital video camera. I wanted Sandy to speak to the children. She would not."

In her final days, Sandy was in tremendous pain. She had a collapsed vertebra. "She had no bones left," Bob says. But she did not want to let go. And all he could do was urge the therapist they were seeing, "Please, tell Sandy to quit, that it's time to die." When she was about to die, she asked to be put on a respirator. "I refused," he says. "Because it was futile."

Is he bitter and angry? Bob says he is not. But he does wish he could grasp the meaning of Sandy's death. "I have wondered all my life about God's grand plan for our lives. I keep asking God. He doesn't talk to me."

HELPING YOUR WIFE PREPARE

At the very least, a couple needs to follow the practical advice that social worker Patricia Spicer gives. There are some "hot button" issues that should be addressed, she notes. Is your will up to date? Does the husband have power of attorney? Is he the designated health-care proxy?

If your wife wants to discuss her death, don't cut her off. It may be very important for her to share her wishes. Does she want cremation or burial? Who should get her favorite bracelet?

Then there are the deeper emotional issues. If you and your wife have children, she may want to leave them a legacy and not know how to do that.

When a breast cancer patient is nearing death, and she and her husband have kids, nurse Lillie Shockney tells the husband to go to a greeting card store at the nearest mall and buy a batch for their children—a card for every birthday until the kids turn 21, cards for Christmas, for graduation, for a wedding, for the birth of a child. If the cards are not on display, she says, ask the manager to look in the stockroom. Then your wife can, if she wishes, write a message on each card. Keep the stash of cards in a lockbox, Shockney suggests, so they don't get lost or damaged.

When the children read those cards as the years go by, they will feel the presence of their mother, they will see her handwriting, they will receive her wishes and wisdom.

The very act of writing those cards, and of leaving other messages, can be therapeutic. After she was diagnosed with metastatic disease, Jay Grogan's wife, Lynn, bought copies of *The Alchemist*, a fable about the importance of following your dreams, to leave for her two sons. In each copy, she made notes in the margin about why she loved the book. "*The Alchemist* was almost a life lesson to her," Jay says. "She wanted them to have this life lesson."

When Lynn died, her sons were ages 12 and 9. She knew they would have a confirmation ceremony at 13, and she wrote each one a letter telling them why the confirmation was important, and "here's what I would have told you if I was there." Jay kept the letters tucked in a safe until the time came.

Jay didn't even know Lynn was doing this at first. When I spoke to him, she'd been gone 3 years, and he told me, "I still find stuff, little notes she'd leave. 'Dear Trent and Reed . . . I know this was your favorite book. When you run into this, there's no telling how long it's been since I've gone.' "

But as with just about every issue in breast cancer, there is no right or wrong way to handle an impending death. Your wife may find comfort in writing messages or in making videotapes. Or, like Larry Gold's* wife, she may not want to leave letters or tapes behind. "She thought about it, but she didn't want to be frozen on a piece of paper," he says. "She wanted the kids to have living memories of her." That would be Larry's task, to remind his three daughters of who their mother was and how she loved them and shaped their lives.

WHEN DEATH COMES

No one can tell you how you will react when your wife dies.

In fact, your reaction may puzzle or dismay you. Jay Grogan was surprised that when Lynn died, he was "not all weepy or upset." He felt guilty that he didn't feel worse. And he told a buddy from Australia how upset he was that he wasn't more . . . upset.

"Jay, what you are talking about? You did that a long time ago," his friend said. "I remember when Lynn was diagnosed, you were unreachable for a week. You did your grieving back then. You might have had a little left to do, but not that much." His friend's theory is that each individual has a finite amount of grief within for a loved one. It might be a huge amount, but it is not boundless. When that loved one dies, you must grieve that finite amount. You grieve until there's no more grieving to be done.

Jay recognized the truth in his friend's theory. "I did as much grieving in the 2 or 3 days after Lynn was diagnosed with metastatic disease as I did at any point in the process, including the moment of her death."

When that moment does come, then you are no longer a breast cancer husband. You are a breast cancer widower. "Watching her go—it was as if there was an invisible hand on a dimmer switch," says Steve Bean, 60, of Exeter, New Hampshire, whose wife, Marion, died 2 years ago. "Every day, the light in her eyes went slowly out until she faded away right before my eyes. The house is very big now, for just me. I am rattling around in it like a BB in a boxcar."

As Jay Grogan learned, the process of mourning is highly individual. "I cried every night for weeks," says Bob Marovich, remembering his wife's death from breast cancer 4 years ago. "You're at home and you open up a drawer and find something of hers, and that'll pretty much knock you out for the entire evening.

"The grief is always tucked away somewhere," he adds. But as the years have gone by, he has come to see that "there is light at the end of the tunnel. It's not a permanent black cloud over you. Every day it gets a little easier. Eventually you get to thinking of the things about your wife that made you laugh, or you'll say 'if she had seen this, she would have been miffed.'"

A grief therapist might be able to help you come to terms with the range of your emotions. After Linda McCartney died of breast cancer in 1998, husband Paul McCartney told the British newspaper *The Sun* that he sought help from a therapist. When his wife passed away, Paul said that he was beset by feelings of guilt. He wished he had been the perfect husband for Linda, and, of course, no one can be perfect all of the time. Talking to the therapist helped him comes to terms with his grief—and his guilt.

Lillie Shockney, who has been my inspiration and guide throughout this book, and who seems to have a suggestion for every dilemma that faces a breast cancer husband, has one more suggestion to help a husband prepare for his lonely life after his wife is gone. It is an awkward suggestion to include in this book, because it is not something that she tells the husbands. Still, I think it is important to pass on her thought. When she meets a couple, and the woman is likely to die from breast cancer because there's not much the doctors can do, Lillie tries to speak to someone else in the family—the woman's sister, perhaps, or a dear friend. She tells that person to buy a card for the wife, so she can write a note to her husband for him to read after she is gone.

In it, Lillie hopes the wife will tell him, "I hope you have moved on." In other words, it's okay to love again.

TIPS ➢ ➢ ➢

1. Consider seeing a therapist sooner rather than later. Talking about your feelings as you care for your wife in her dying days may make it easier for you to cope when the inevitable comes to pass.
2. Don't make your wife feel badly about being dependent on you. When Janie Goldman was fighting cancer symptoms, her husband, Mike, had to learn to take her arm subtly to keep her from tripping, and not to say anything that would make her feel bad about her dependence.
3. Walking in a breast cancer event in your wife's memory, setting up a fund for research in her name—these are some of the ways that a breast cancer husband can keep his wife's spirit alive.

➢ BONUS TIP

Maybe your wife won't want to talk about her funeral, but maybe she will. Bob Marovich's wife, Pat, was a school music teacher and planned the music for her own service. "We want to make this right for you," a musician told her. "Don't do it for *me*," Pat said with a laugh. "I'm going to be dead."

The New Normal

Breast cancer survivors—and their mates—face an unfamiliar future

In opera, it ain't over 'til the fat lady sings.

Yogi Berra famously said, "It ain't over till it's over."

And breast cancer, well, the truth is that it's never truly over, although husbands sure would like to think it is.

BACK TO WHAT?

When a woman's active treatment ends, many a guy will toss the car keys to his wife and say, "Okay, honey, you're back on carpool duty. When you do the laundry, make sure you iron my white dress shirt. Oh, and by the way, we're out of milk."

I'm exaggerating . . . but only a little. Speaking of the post-treatment period, psychologist and breast cancer survivor Janet Reibstein, an American who teaches at the University of Exeter in England, observes, "Even the best men don't get it right all the time. One of the ways they don't is that they really want you to be okay. And if you are looking good and competent, they think you are good. But you are not over it. You go up and down."

"My husband was truly a saint," says Carole O'Toole, 48. "He never missed an appointment." But when she had her last treatment, he said, "It's behind us now." Carole remembers her surprise—and anger. "I said, 'I have to live with this every day for the rest of my life. It's not something you can just close the door on or wrap up in a box and say it's gone.'"

You and your wife are entering a new phase of life. In the world of breast cancer, this period is known as the New Normal. No matter how much you yearn for the Old Normal, the theory goes, you can never go back to your life exactly the way it was.

Part of the New Normal is that breast cancer is now a member of your family. At times (and as more time goes by), the disease may fade from your mind, like a distant relative you really don't care for. But you cannot rush the process. "You can talk yourself to death, but you can't make it happen faster than it's going to happen," says Bethesda, Maryland, psychologist Venus Masselam, Ph.D. "You can't make yourself feel more secure than you're going to feel."

A change of scene, however, could at least give you a break. Marsha finished radiation in May. We went on vacation in late June. Getting away from the cancer reminders in every corner of the house—from upcoming appointments marked on the calendar to the jar of Astroglide in the medicine chest—was uplifting in ways I couldn't have imagined. We spent a lazy day in a small Vermont town, and when the sun was setting, I turned to Marsha and said, "We didn't talk about breast cancer today." And we looked at each other, astonished, because we hadn't had a respite from breast cancer talk since Marsha was first diagnosed some 10 months earlier.

But even when the memories have begun to recede, there will be moments when breast cancer comes roaring back—perhaps on the eve of a checkup with one of your wife's cancer docs, or when the disease claims a victim from your circle of friends or even from the world of celebrities.

DIFFERENT SPEEDS

It is only natural that the breast cancer husband moves forward at a faster pace than his wife.

First of all, she may be bone tired and he's not. "Fatigue is the number one side effect," says Marisa Weiss, M.D., the Philadelphia breast radiation oncologist who founded the Web site breastcancer.org. Her patients sometimes say they feel as if they've aged 100 years in 6 months of treatment. And it may take another 6 months to recover their energy. The fatigue may stem from shock, stress, fear, anxiety, and depression—not to mention the cumulative toll of chemotherapy and hot flashes that interrupt a good night's sleep. "Patients move like robots from one treatment to the next," Dr. Weiss explains. "They don't have a chance to come up for air. They may feel worn down at the end of this whole process." Your wife may also feel worn down from aches and pains that result from treatment—or that are brought on by hormonal therapies. Those estrogen-blocking pills might also affect her mood and disposition. So can the abrupt entry into menopause that chemo can trigger.

What's more, the husband's body does not continually remind him of breast cancer. His wife's does. She looks in the mirror at a reconstructed breast, or at no breast at all, or at a breast with a dent from a lumpectomy. She still has a numb spot under her arm months after the axillary dissection. Or if she feels a back pain she's never felt before, she may worry that the disease has crept into her bones. If your wife is thinking about breast cancer and you're not, you might be tempted to tell her she's fine and to put those thoughts out of her mind.

Remember way back when, in the early days just after diagnosis, she may have been in a deep breast cancer funk and you tried to cheer her up—which only made her feel as if she didn't have the right to feel bad? You'll need to be just as sensitive in the post-treatment phase. Tell your wife, "I understand how you feel." (And what she's feeling, by the way, is normal. There are times when anxiety spikes for cancer patients, and one of them is at the end of treatment.) Then you can gently remind her of encouraging words the doctor has said or of the fact that every day she goes without a recurrence is another day that she's a breast cancer survivor—and that the further out from diagnosis a patient is, the less likely it is that the cancer will come back.

If 2 years have gone by from the date of surgery and your wife has no sign of cancer, then she has passed through the period with the highest risk of recurrence. Five years is another milestone to mark. After 7½ years, if a cancer is found in the breast, it is considered a new breast cancer.

But the threat of metastatic disease lingers on. "Do you use the word 'cure' for breast cancer patients?" I asked one oncologist. "Um, yeah, cautiously," the doctor hedged. "There are people who live their full lives without breast cancer coming back." Then she told the sad truth about the disease: "Once you die of something else, you know you've been cured of breast cancer."

So that's why your wife is worried.

WHAT, NO DOCS?

One of the strangest things about the New Normal is that your wife may actually miss the days when she was in treatment. She surely won't miss the needles and the side effects and the inconvenience and the drain on her energy and time. But she may miss the idea that she is actively fighting cancer. Taking tamoxifen or another anticancer pill every day is part of the ongoing battle, but it's not the same as frequent visits to a team of knowledgeable, confidence-inspiring doctors who take her blood pressure and test her blood and make sure everything is all right.

When active treatment was over, my wife definitely felt as if she'd been cut adrift. She would see her team of docs—the surgeon, the radiologist, the oncologist, and the radiation oncologist—every 3 months for the first year. Then every 6 months for the second year. And then once a year. They would ask her about any changes in her health, they would draw blood to check for proteins that are a sign of cancer, they would do mammograms and palpate her breasts.

But there would be no monthly or even yearly scans in search of metastatic breast cancer.

This absolutely floored my wife. Many other women are equally nonplussed. What—no scans? No hunt for those microscopic cancer cells? The problem is that high-tech scans would uncover all sorts of spots and specks that would turn out to be false alarms. There'd be too much information. And if a metastasis were uncovered, well, there's not a lot of difference between

(continued on page 279)

LESSENING THE RISK OF LYMPHEDEMA

One more reason they call breast cancer the gift that keeps on giving: In addition to lingering post-chemo side effects and worries about recurrence, there's the low but lifelong threat of lymphedema for women who have had lymph nodes removed from an armpit.

You can be forgiven if you don't know exactly what lymphedema is. Perhaps your wife's surgeon explained the condition, and your wife (and you) forgot all about it. That's understandable, given the circumstances. Or maybe the surgeon never said a word. That happens, too.

Lymphedema is the medical term for swelling caused by an accumulation of lymphatic fluid in tissue. I like the way physical therapist Janet Sobel explains the affliction. Start by thinking of the rush-hour traffic at Bradley Boulevard and Wisconsin Avenue, Sobel says—that's a major intersection near her home in Chevy Chase, Maryland. "Bumper to bumper" would be an apt description. Now imagine the traffic if a lane were shut down because of construction. You'd have a parking lot.

In the human body, the lymph nodes are akin to the traffic lanes. They are the vessels that carry lymphatic fluid through the body. A woman has about 700 lymph nodes in all, and about 35 to 40 in each armpit. When checking the nodes for cancer, the surgeon may remove just one or two—the sentinel nodes that would probably be affected first by a spreading cancer—or a larger batch. The more nodes cut out (especially if the number is greater than seven), the harder it may be for lymphatic fluid to drain properly. In other words, the surgeon is taking out a traffic lane. (The good news is that you have many more traffic lanes in your armpit than there are on most major highways.)

When a body's fluid traffic is normal, the missing lymph nodes probably won't cause any problems. But a skin wound, an insect bite, or even a sunburn on the arm in question can cause the lymphatic system to rev up in defense—and that can lead to a backup of fluid. Although stories circulate of sudden and severe swelling, the swelling is likely to start slowly. If your wife (or you) see a slight puffiness, or if the bones on her hand seem a little less prominent, she should drink lots of water and pay close attention to the swelling.

If the swelling worsens, or if there

is a sign of infection—if the arm is red or warm to the touch, or your wife is running a fever—that's the time to call whichever of her doctors seems most tuned in to lymphedema. An infection "is considered an emergency," stresses Philadelphia breast radiation oncologist Marisa Weiss, M.D., and your wife should visit the emergency room if necessary. The next step is to see a physical therapist certified in lymphedema management, who may be able to reverse the swelling. Your wife can ask for names from her cancer docs or, if she's in a support group, from her breast cancer circle. Or contact the nearest breast cancer center for suggestions.

Breast cancer survivors with lymphedema may suffer physical pain in the arm as well as psychological pain. If the swelling is plainly seen, they might be embarrassed to wear sleeveless tops; they sometimes must wrap the arm in a flesh-colored elasticized sleeve or in bandages to manage the condition.

Once a woman is diagnosed with lymphedema, she has it for life. If treatment is effective, her arm may look normal, with only occasional bouts of swelling. Other women always have some degree of swelling.

The risk of lymphedema among women who've had lymph nodes removed ranges from 5 to 25 percent, depending on the nature of the patient's treatment. Taking out a lot of lymph nodes and adding a heap of chemo drugs will increase the risk. Radiation increases the risk a little; it causes scarring that can block lymphatic flow. As more women have the sentinel node biopsy, which takes far fewer lymph nodes from the underarm than a full dissection would, the number of new cases should decline. But even a sentinel node procedure could put a woman at risk for lymphedema.

To help your wife reduce her risk, start nudging:

1. Before a doctor's visit, remind your wife that taking blood pressure or blood draws from the arm in question is not advisable. The tightness of the cuff puts stress on the arm; the needle prick creates a break in the skin. If a woman has had lymph nodes removed from both armpits, she may want to offer her foot for blood draws and leg for blood pressure, or at least alternate arms.

(continued)

LESSENING THE RISK OF LYMPHEDEMA (CONT.)

2. Remind her to avoid wearing constrictive sleeves or jewelry, especially when flying. (Air travel does not appear to cause lymphedema, although it can aggravate pre-existing edema.)
3. Tell her to guzzle 6 to 8 glasses of water every day.
4. Tell her to drink even more if she's flying (and to avoid salty snacks).
5. Encourage her to exercise. Lifting weights is fine, as long as your wife starts at a low weight—say, 1 to 4 pounds—and gradually works her way up to heavier weights, using her arm's response as a guide to whether she is ready to progress. Good muscle tone is helpful to the normal flow of the lymphatic system.
6. Do the really heavy lifting for her. It's fine for your wife to lift stuff, but she should stay away from objects much heavier than she's used to—say, a suitcase for an upcoming trip. If she's traveling solo, spring for a suitcase with wheels.
7. Remind her not to carry a shoulder bag or grocery bags with the at-risk arm. Better yet, bring in the groceries yourself.
8. Buy a tube of an antibiotic ointment like Neosporin and Band-Aids with built-in antiobiotic ointment for your wife to keep in her purse (and a set for the medicine chest at home). If she gets a scratch or a bug bite on the vulnerable arm, remind her to apply the antibiotic ointment.
9. Bug her about posture: Standing up straight is a boon to the lymphatic system and also keeps the chest wall open.
10. Bug spray and gloves are musts in the garden, oven mitts in the kitchen.
11. Biting or picking at fingernails is a bad idea.
12. Well-moisturized skin is less likely to have cracks that let in bacteria. So buy your wife some nice lotion and then rub it in, especially after a shower or bath.

Above all, don't dismiss your wife's fears of lymphedema. And if she develops the condition? Janet Sobel has asked her patients what they think breast cancer husbands should know about living with lymphedema. "The most common answer was that the husband might get used to seeing the lymphedema, but the woman *never* gets used to it," Sobel says. "It affects how she feels, what she can wear, and is a constant reminder of the cancer."

finding it in a scan and finding it based on a report of symptoms (headache, backache, and so on). All the doctors can do is try their best to manage the symptoms, beat the cancer into remission, and hope they can keep the patient healthy for a long time.

As for the blood tests, they have their defenders and detractors in the medical community. A clean blood test is indeed reassuring for the patient—but it doesn't guarantee that she is cancer free. "You also have to consider the anxiety caused not just by an elevated blood marker, but by all of the tests that may be needed to try to find out where the increased marker is coming from" is the cautionary note on breastcancer.org. And even if the blood tests were to signal a metastatic recurrence, at this time, the patient does not gain better odds of survival by finding out sooner rather than later.

What can you tell your wife to help her cope with the uncertainty of a life where cancer might (or might not) recur? My wife's oncologist, Fred Smith, M.D., who practices in Chevy Chase, Maryland, had excellent advice. I think of his words just about every day. You could spend the rest of your days worrying about the possibility of a recurrence, he told Marsha. If you never have a recurrence, you've wasted all that time worrying. And if you do have a recurrence, you've still wasted all that time worrying when you could have been enjoying life.

So we try not to worry. We don't always succeed. But we keep trying. I also keep in mind the remarks of a breast cancer husband whose wife had several healthy years after her treatment, but then suffered a recurrence and died of the disease: "Maybe I should have been a bigger fan of denial." Not to deny what had happened, he explained, but to deny breast cancer the power to cast a shadow over their lives during the years when she was feeling okay.

Your wife can quell her anxiety in various ways. She doesn't have control over cancer, but she does have control over scheduling. When her doctor visits go from every 3 months to every 6 months to once a year, you might suggest that she set up appointments so she's seeing one of her docs every couple of months rather than seeing them all the same week, then waiting a year for the next go-round.

And you might take a lesson from Irene Gage, M.D., my wife's radiation oncologist.

At one of Marsha's visits, about a year after radiation had been completed, Dr. Gage asked a few medical questions—any coughing, shortness of breath, morning headaches, bone pain, breast pain? Then she posed questions that had nothing to do with spotting a recurrence. She wanted to know how Marsha feels about coming in for checkups: "Does it make you anxious? Is it a good moment or a bad moment?"

What profoundly human questions. "In a lot of ways, a new process starts after treatment ends," Dr. Gage explains. "I'm trying to get a sense of where somebody is in that process. I think that for some women, doctor's visits are reassuring, and for some women, they're very upsetting. My line is that if we cure the cancer and lose the patient, we only get partial credit." Not every doctor will bring up the topic. But you can. Go ahead, ask your wife how she's feeling about her checkups. (Of course, you probably already have a good idea—many husbands told me they could tell when a doctor's visit was looming, because their wives would become irritable or depressed.) Then ask her if there's anything you can do to help.

One husband told me that he goes with his wife to her follow-ups whenever he can. "If she were ever to hear bad news, I'd want to be there with her," he said. I've gone a few times with Marsha, and I heartily endorse the idea of continuing to be your wife's appointment pal. There's really no downside. Your wife will know that you care. Plus, those waiting room magazines are just the best!

You can also try to build in a nice outing to go along with the visit. Meet your wife for the appointment, then take her to lunch afterward. Or plan something special that night. At least then she'll have a good association with her cancer checkups: a glass of wine, a grilled chicken Caesar salad, and thou.

WHAT IF . . .

The big fear in just about every patient's mind (and in the minds of husbands, too) is that the cancer will come back. Local or regional recurrence—another tumor in the breast or cancer cells in the lymph nodes—would be bad enough. Systemic recurrence—cancer that has spread to other parts of the body—would seem catastrophic.

When couples get the news that breast cancer has made an unwelcome return, they typically have that deer-in-the-headlights look. As if they've been sucker punched, said a breast cancer husband who has seen the expression on the faces of a couple or two in a support group he attends.

Here we go again.

A newly discovered tumor in either breast is eminently treatable. If the tumor occurs in a breast that's had a lumpectomy and radiation, then the option is almost certainly going to be a mastectomy. Doctors don't like to do a second round of radiation, and thus a second lumpectomy is not advisable. The surgeon will try to remove the cancer, if possible. If a new lesion is found in the opposite breast, then the surgical option will depend on the circumstances, just as it did the first time around.

If your wife is diagnosed with metastatic disease, then she is entering a new arena of breast cancer. The goal is to knock the disease into remission and manage the symptoms. Your wife could have a decade or more ahead of her. Or a year or less. The chapter Mysteries of Metastatic Disease on page 246 will give you some idea of the unpredictability of a metastasis—and the bravery of the women (and their husbands) who live with this burden.

BRAIN FREEZE, HOT FLASHES

To add to post-treatment anxiety, breast cancer patients who've undergone chemotherapy may feel as if the chemo cocktail has shaken up their bodies and minds.

You may have heard your wife talk about "chemo brain." If you haven't heard the phrase by now . . . well, maybe you've heard it and you just don't remember. Because even husbands have a touch of memory lapse after the stress of cancer. They say it takes two—husband and wife—to recollect all the details of a year fighting cancer, and that's no joke.

Docs talk about how breast cancer survivors may have trouble with "cognitive functions." And that would be . . . ¿ "Memory and the ability to think clearly and to know where you put the keys," explains Dr. Weiss. In other words, your wife might not be able to juggle tasks like she used to. "Chemo brain is not dementia," emphasizes Ian Tannock, M.D., professor of medical oncology at the University of Toronto's Princess Margaret Hospital, who is studying the phenomenon. "It's subtle. It's not something you would notice in normal conversation."

Doctors have come up with various theories to explain the post-treatment memory problems that afflict 15 to 30 percent of chemotherapy patients. Anxiety blocks memory in a major way, so forgetfulness could be a reaction to the stress of diagnosis and treatment. Women in menopause report similar memory lapses, so some oncologists think that the chemo push into menopause may be the cause. Or it could just be the normal result of aging and of having too much to do. Dr. Tannock, however, points to some half a dozen recent studies pitting chemo patients against a control group: the chemo patients showed more evidence of impairment. "I think there is enough evidence to suggest a separate effect for chemotherapy," he says, although it's not yet known exactly how the drugs might affect the brain's ability to function, or how long the cognitive impairment will last.

In any event, no one's saying that chemo brain is a figment of the woman's imagination. And no husband should be dismissive or rude when his wife complains that she doesn't have the same ability to juggle at work or when she forgets about Johnny's karate class or she can't remember where she left the keys.

But that doesn't mean it won't be a little unnerving.

Barbara Dorand, 50, of Pike Road, Alabama, used to be able to memorize the telephone directory, her husband, Rodney, says. After chemo, she'd tell him to do something, and he'd do it. The next day, she'd ask him to do the chore again. He finally got his son and daughter to testify in his behalf. Not to make his wife feel bad, but just to show her that he wasn't exaggerating when he said, "You already told me that."

If your wife seems to be suffering from chemo brain, she'll need to devise ways to compensate. Writing notes to herself can help. You can help, too. Check the calendar (digital or paper) where your family logs appointments so you can remind her—in a subtle, not condescending way—about the daily agenda. "Looks like the kids have their piano lessons today" ought to do it.

Hot flashes may enter your wife's (and your) life, as well. That's another menopausal by-product, courtesy of chemo. She might suffer from night

GUY TALK

"I wanted to believe that everything was over, and we could get back to normal. And that certainly wasn't the case."

—JEFF ZITELMAN, 49
Kensington, Maryland

sweats, or a hot feeling in her scalp and face that spreads to her neck and body. She could be drenched in sweat, then chilled a minute later. The flashes result from the body's resetting of its thermostat. Symptoms typically resolve themselves in a few years, but tamoxifen might exacerbate them. Husbands might exacerbate them, too, if they're short on sympathy. So be a sport. "My wife is always turning up the air-conditioning," says Claude Robinson, 72, of Capitol Heights, Maryland. "Last night it was cool out, 66 degrees, and she's hot. What do you do? I got a blanket."

Then there is the matter of weight gain. Studies show that women tend to add at least a few—and sometimes many—pounds during chemotherapy. They may be less active during treatment, and, if they were pre- or perimenopausal before chemo, their metabolism will most likely have slowed down after they were pushed into menopause. The new menopausal metabolism doesn't bode well for losing the weight, either. Tamoxifen gets the blame a lot of the time, just as it does for vaginal dryness. Studies indicate comparable weight gain in women on tamoxifen and women of the same age who aren't taking the drug. But tamoxifen could still be making your wife hungrier than she was before cancer.

Many women have told me about the phenomenon of ravenous hunger. "I could eat shoes," says still-svelte Carol Stevenson. My wife agrees. She met with a nutritionist who gave her all kinds of helpful advice: mini-meals, more protein, no snacks while reading the Sunday paper. None of the strategies seemed to make her significantly less hungry. She met with a personal trainer who specializes in breast cancer patients, and who pushed her to exercise a little harder. In the end, she did shed a few of the extra pounds, but she also had to make her peace with a new baseline weight. The empty pit in her stomach isn't quite as bottomless as it was right after she finished chemo and radiation, but about a third of the time she still feels a gnawing hunger.

What this means for the breast cancer husband is that you will almost certainly be asked the question that all men dread: "Do I look fat?" I've learned that "Compared to what?" is not a good answer. The best reply is, "I love you no matter what" or "I always think you're beautiful"—an assurance that you do not love your wife any less after cancer.

But I think there's room for a measure of honesty. If your wife is asking whether she looks fat in a particular garment, ask her if she wants the unvarnished truth. If she says "yes," give her your assessment. My wife really does want to know if a dress or sweater makes her appear slim or bulky. So I gird my loins and I tell her. (And Marsha, dear, if you're reading this chapter, you look great! Really!)

If your wife is dismayed by the extra pounds (and if you're carrying around a few more than you should), perhaps the two of you can make a diet/exercise pact together. Keep in mind that this is not just a matter of vanity for your wife. A study presented this year at the American Association for Cancer Research found that breast cancer survivors who walked just 1 to 3 hours a week, at the far from Olympian pace of 3 mph, improved their chances of survival compared to sedentary breast cancer survivors (perhaps because the walkers burn up fat that would otherwise produce estrogen, which can promote the growth of breast cancer). More strenuous exercise reduced the risk of dying from breast cancer even more.

HEY, BIG SPENDER

The New Normal isn't just about coping with the specter of cancer as well as lingering side effects. It's also about enjoying every day. For many couples, this leads to what women jokingly call "the tumor upgrade." In other words, retail therapy.

"Breast cancer is an expensive disease," one woman told me, and she wasn't referring to doctor's bills. Even the most frugal couples (and I think my wife and I qualify on that count) may find that they are a little more free-spending after a brush with cancer. Sure, it's great to save for retirement and college tuitions and the new roof you'll need someday, but cancer may convince you that it's just as important to treat yourself well in the present.

That's how my wife got her breast cancer car.

We were sitting on the porch one fine Sunday in August, a couple of months after Marsha's treatment had ended. We were a one-car family (a sensible Toyota Camry) and were planning to buy a second car, a used one, because our older daughter was about to get her driver's license. As my wife perused the Sunday paper, she looked at Toyota ads and said, "You know, we can get a new Prius, the hybrid that gets sensational gas mileage, for just a little more than we'd have to spend for a used Toyota or Honda."

The next thing I knew, we were at the dealership, test-driving a Prius and then signing on the dotted line, no money down, 5 years of payments.

Marsha loves her zippy, gas-conserving car. So do I, whenever she lets me drive it.

(P.S. I still haven't told her about the breast cancer husband I talked to who bought his wife a new sports car.)

Guys deserve a treat, too. Hey, you were a good caregiver. Go ahead, knock yourself out! When I phoned breast cancer husband Colton Young of Chalfont, Pennsylvania, his wife, Kathleen McCarthy, answered the phone. I could hear someone banging away on the drums in the background. I asked if it was their son. It turned out to be Colton.

"I've played sporadically for about the last 10 years, and I've played seriously now for about the last 20 months," says Colton, 42. When Kathleen, who was diagnosed with breast cancer at age 36, finished her treatment, "she got the furniture she always wanted, I got my drums. I mean, it's a nice set, new drums, with cymbals and everything. We bought things, but we didn't buy them impulsively. These are things we knew we were going to get eventually. I said, 'You know what? Now is good. We can afford it, we're not going into debt. Let's get it now. We've been through a lot. If we can garner a few smiles via material possessions, let's do it.'"

Kathleen gets some smiles, too—when Colton takes a break from the drums.

WHAT NEXT, MY LOVE?

That's the question that you and your wife may be facing. For some people, the New Normal isn't simply a place where you spend money more freely.

It's a stage of life where you and your wife may follow dreams you've long had, or find out how much you mean to each other. "I never knew how much I loved and needed my wife," says actor Michael Tucker. "It's just a damn shame we need a two-by-four across the chops before we realize this."

Indeed, many breast cancer couples report that their marriages have deepened, with both partners feeling a renewed appreciation and more heartfelt love for each other. "It gave me more confidence in my marriage," says breast cancer survivor Leni English, 41, of Makawao, Hawaii. "Because Glen was just very supportive." Glen agrees—he took 2 weeks off from work to care for his wife after her mastectomy. "Doing things for her and helping her," he says, "made our marriage stronger."

Some therapists half-joke that when breast cancer survivors talk about the way their lives have changed for the better, listeners say, "I'd sure like to get some of what they got."

Take it from my wife: No, you wouldn't. Really. As one woman told Karen Weihs, M.D., a professor of psychiatry and behavioral sciences at George Washington University, "Breast cancer isn't a growth experience, it's a growth." But for some women (and their husbands), the disease can indeed be both a trauma and an opportunity for positive changes in their lives.

There are three human responses to any traumatic event, says Tzipi Weiss, Ph.D., visiting assistant professor at Long Island University, C.W. Post campus, who has studied couples to see how they weather a trauma like breast cancer.

Couples can deteriorate into dysfunctionality. They can return to their previous level of functioning. Or they can move to a different way of life that seems to be an improvement over their previous existence—that's what Dr. Weiss calls "post-traumatic growth," a term that describes the stories you hear of women whose breast cancer was a catalyst for finding a new career or a new hobby or maybe just a newfound appreciation for the beauties of the world.

The idea that pain and suffering can lead to enlightenment is not new. "It's been in our civilization for thousands of years," says Dr. Weiss. But in this age of the short attention span, trauma victims may feel pressure from family and friends to get over it and move on. Post-traumatic growth, however, will occur only if you take the opposite stance—if you reflect on what has happened, including the bad and the ugly, and look for new possibilities in the future. In Dr. Weiss's research, 96 percent of breast cancer survivors report positive changes in their lives. It doesn't matter what stage the cancer was. If the woman was at stage 0 but feels she has undergone a major life trauma, then she has the potential for growth.

As for breast cancer husbands—we surely haven't suffered as much as our wives, but many of us have gone along for the cancer ride. Because we, too, have been affected by the disease, the National Cancer Institute includes us in the definition of "breast cancer survivor." But what do we get out of it? Just a drum set? Or something deeper and more profound?

"The potential for pain and gain is shared by the marital partners," Dr. Weiss believes. Maybe your wife is serving as a model for you. Or maybe you're a model for her. Linda and Allen Anderson of Minneapolis both report the same kind of new feelings. "Life is so much more precious," says Linda, 58, who had four surgeries after her January 2002 diagnosis: two lumpectomies that didn't result in clear margins, then a mastectomy, then reconstruction. "Little things mean so much"—like taking walks with her husband. "You learn from everything that comes in life," says Allen, 50. "My love for Linda is deeper now." Linda adds that going through breast cancer treatment has shown her how strong she can be, "and the knowledge of that strength is a gift for the rest of your life."

Frank Sadowski would agree that life has changed, and not in bad ways. At age 45, his wife, Laura, had a mastectomy and "3½ months of really tough chemo." Now they are forging their New Normal. "Cancer certainly isn't a gift," says Sadowski, the vice president for consumer electronics merchandising at amazon.com. "But it's a blessing."

He reflects on his choice of words. "As crazy as that sounds coming out of my mouth, I think, in a way, it has been a blessing . . . for my wife, and for both of us, in different ways. It has really changed her outlook on life. She enjoys the things she enjoys more. She has lots fewer strings attached to her life. She doesn't enjoy things conditionally or intellectually as before. She just enjoys things."

When we spoke, the family was getting ready for a trip to Maui. "This is a woman who has never spent any money," he says. "We are far from fabulously wealthy, but we have been doing well for quite a few years. And I could not get her to spend any money on herself." Frank is happy that now she'll go out and buy stuff that makes her happy. She'll go get a massage and not worry about forking over $80 for a 45-minute rubdown. She won't spy a $100 dress and say "I could make it for $10." She'll just buy it. "If it's something you enjoy, just enjoy," he recommends.

The change isn't just about material things. "For me, I wouldn't say I feel like it's been a radical change," he says, "like getting hit on the head by a coconut or seeing God next to you. But there's been a significant change in the way I prioritize things and what I think is important.

"Things that used to be really, really important to me, like problems at work, aren't important in the same way. Life's too short to mess around with this stuff." In the past he would have worried about workplace problems. Now, he says, "I don't have time to worry about that."

Overall, women do tend to report "post-traumatic growth" more often than their husbands do. Maybe that's because they're more willing to wrestle with their negative emotions, says Dr. Weiss. And that can put them on a pathway to growth. We husbands . . . well, what can I say? We're experts at denial.

The feeling of positive change can fade as the years go by. So does growth erode with time? "I think what it means," says Dr. Weiss, "is as you get further away from the illness, you define yourself less and less by the illness." The wife doesn't want to be identified solely as a "cancer survivor." And the husband doesn't want to be known as a "breast cancer husband" for the rest of his life. The more time that passes after diagnosis and treatment, the less anxious your wife may be about dying, and the less nervous you may be. Both of you may begin thinking more like the rest of the world—you know, that you'll never meet the Grim Reaper.

But maybe you'll be fortunate enough to make a change that can improve the quality of your lives for years to come.

Gary and Becky Krimstein both held impossibly demanding jobs in local television production when she was diagnosed with breast cancer 6 years ago. She was 35 at the time. After her lumpectomy and radiation and four rounds of chemo, they thought about the dreams they wanted to pursue. As Gary says, "We don't want to wait for tomorrow to do them."

Change isn't easy, and the Maryland couple quickly slipped back into old routines. They weren't happy about that turn of events. "We were, like, there are so many great things we should be doing, why are we in the jobs we have and not seeing each other more? Why are we spending so much time at work?"

They knew all the conventional wisdom about downshifting from high-pressure but high-paying jobs—you can't take a cut in salary, you can't give up good benefits. Five years after Becky's diagnosis, they decided to make changes anyway. They left their chaotic lifestyle behind and pursued their goal of starting their own video production business. The childless workaholics do have more time together. A great deal of that time was spent working on a documentary about Becky's breast cancer experience: *A Cancer Rainbow: Snapshots from My Journey.* Their film has aired on PBS stations and won a gold medal at the New York International Video and Film Festival.

"I would not trade the time we had working together for anything," Gary says. "It's been . . . "

And Becky, a sweet-faced redhead, finishes his sentence, in the time-honored tradition of couples: ". . . good."

When I look up from my notebook, I see that Gary is crying a little. Becky is, too. And I can feel tears welling up in my eyes, too.

I guess that's what they mean by post-traumatic growth.

THE PINK RIBBON WANTS YOU

One very concrete way that women change their lives is to become activists for breast cancer. There is an army of women, many of them breast cancer survivors and many of them family and friends of survivors (and victims), who devote untold hours to the cause. They raise money, they speak out, they volunteer for help lines, they "race for the cure." They might even spend 2 or 3 days walking and sleeping in tents in all kinds of awful weather, from pouring rain to late spring sleet to blistering heat.

Husbands react to this activism in different ways. They may be proud, but they may also worry that it's too much breast cancer. After Cookie Medansky had been volunteering for the Y-ME breast cancer hotline for a decade, her husband, Earl, could see that the work was getting her down. So he asked her to back off. "After 50 years together, a certain amount of time we listen to each other, but most of the time we don't," Earl says with a laugh. But Cookie did listen this time. "And since she's backed off, it's been better," Earl says. "Ten years was enough."

"I completely support her advocacy work," says John Salamone, whose wife, Jeanine, volunteers for the Young Survival Coalition. "It's a chance to help so many people, to make a difference. But our bedroom is our sanctuary—do we have to look at Young Survival Coalition stuff in our bedroom?"

There were times when Bob Strickland used to wish his wife, Karen, would walk away from her breast cancer volunteer work with the American Cancer Society's Reach to Recovery program. Karen was diagnosed at age 30 in 1984—6 years before they were married. She had a bilateral mastectomy and radiation, and has had various adventures in reconstruction—implants that didn't take, or that sprung a leak. In the summer of 2002, she finished reconstructive surgery using abdominal tissue. So she's had two decades of worry and of activism.

PASS THE BROCCOLI SPROUTS

Next Valentine's Day, instead of giving your wife candy, why not a box of broccoli sprouts?

No, I'm not trying to land you in the doghouse. Broccoli sprouts could turn out to be one of the mightiest cancer-preventers in the garden. In fact, studies have shown them to be an effective weapon against breast tumors, at least ones induced in lab rats.

Over 200 studies have shown that people who eat lots of vegetables have a lower risk of cancer, explains Paul Talalay, M.D., who researches the subject in the department of pharmacology and molecular sciences at the Johns Hopkins School of Medicine in Baltimore. Cruciferous vegetables—which include broccoli, brussels sprouts, cabbage, cauliflower, and kale—are especially helpful. These veggies are rich in sulforaphane, a compound that bolsters the body's natural defenses against cancer-causing chemicals. In a study that Dr. Talalay conducted in 1994, sulforaphane "blocked the formation of mammary tumors in rats treated with a potent carcinogen."

Tests of supermarket broccoli revealed vastly different levels of the protective compound, likely a result of different growing and storage condi-

But now Bob has joined her in the world of breast cancer activism, as one of the relatively few men who walk in the Avon breast cancer events. Bob, 51, is part of the Boston "Men with Heart" contingent—guys whose lives have been touched by the disease and who sign up to trudge a couple of dozen miles to raise money for the cause. In bright yellow T-shirts, they hand out candy and compliments to the female walkers. Although truthfully, the guys get just as many high-fives from women, who are glad to see men who care enough to take part.

"I get an extreme high out of Avon," Bob says—especially the year that a freak May snow-and-sleet storm struck. "We rallied around each other, clung together, and got through the day."

Sounds a lot like going through breast cancer treatment—only Avon provides a well-stocked feeding station every couple of miles.

"I have just been extremely proud of him for doing it and for getting involved," says Karen. "After being involved with the walk, it's like Bob is

---

tions. Broccoli sprouts, however, consistently possess ample quantities of SGS, a sulforaphane precursor.

But is this compound as effective a cancer protector in humans as it is in rodents? Studies are underway.

In the meantime, Dr. Talalay and other Johns Hopkins folks are confident enough to have founded the Brassica Chemoprotection Laboratory, which contracts with farmers to grow the sprouts (with rigorous safeguards to avoid bacterial contamination). Dr. Talalay himself eats an ounce or so of broccoli sprouts two to three times a week—the protective benefit lasts a couple of days, he believes.

You can find a list of supermarkets that carry the sprouts for about $1 an ounce at www.brassica.com. In addition, the Baltimore Coffee and Tea Company, at www.baltcoffee.com, is starting to market tea bags infused with SGS (no, you can't taste the broccoli). The price for 16 teabags is $5 to $6, plus shipping.

So go ahead, toss some broccoli sprouts on your wife's salad or add them to her favorite sandwich. "It can't hurt you," Dr. Talalay says, "and it could benefit you."

Besides, the calorie count is a lot kinder to the waistline than a box of bonbons.

finally a survivor, too. Instead of tagging along with me, he has done something to take control of his feelings in a positive manner." The men who walk the walk agree. The blisters they earn are a kind of self-flagellation—a sign that they, too, have suffered for the cause.

SEEMS LIKE OLD TIMES

The more I talked to people about the New Normal, the more worried I became. I actually kind of liked the Old Normal. I liked our life before cancer came along. Was I an evolutionary throwback? Just another dumb lug who made it to greener pastures and wanted to crawl back to the familiar old mud pit?

It turns out that lots of breast cancer couples yearn for the Old Normal. The Old Normal may have been comfortable for them, says Dr. Gage, my wife's wise radiation oncologist. So they'll try to make the New Normal as much like the Old Normal as they can. "I find that in the people I see, with time it goes back to the Old Normal, particularly if they were happy," says Roz Kleban, the Memorial Sloan-Kettering social worker. If your life wasn't particularly fulfilling, the breast cancer diagnosis may be reason for change. But if you were content with the life you had, there's no reason you shouldn't return to the way things were.

To be sure, Marsha and I had our dreams of big changes after the year of cancer—selling the house, escaping the urban rat race, moving out west to Big Sky country, maybe opening a bed and breakfast (although that would be way too much work, if you ask me).

We didn't make any of those changes.

That's not to say we haven't changed at all. My wife and I never used to talk about tamoxifen, Arimidex, lymphedema, and metastatic disease. We didn't have a house full of T-shirts and hats and pens adorned with pink ribbons. We didn't read every article on breast cancer with extreme interest. As I've mentioned, we're a little more spontaneous in the way we use our hard-earned cash to find some pleasure—although I'd be lying if I said we didn't groan when the credit card bills come in.

Yet despite the changes in our lives, we fell back into many of our old ways and habits. A year after Marsha finished her treatment, she and I were slaving away at the same stressful jobs and griping about the unending parade of chores to do, and grappling with the task of raising two lovely teenage daughters, who occasionally drive their parents a bit batty, as all teenagers do. Sometimes Marsha and I squabble over nothing, like which exit from I-270 will get us home the fastest. (Ha, ha. You were wrong the last time and I was right!) Sometimes we waste a half hour chuckling at a *Seinfeld* rerun we've already seen at least twice before, because thanks to Marsha's chemo brain and my breast cancer husband partial amnesia, all the jokes seem fresh.

Twice a week, when I take out the trash (and grumble about why I'm always the one stuck holding the bag), I might pause to stare up at the big dark sky. Maybe the moon's in view, maybe a few stars are shining. Once in a while, I flash back to those months when surgery loomed, or when chemo ruled our lives, and when the dark nights seemed long and lonely. And then I'm back in the present, stuffing the Hefty bag into the trash can. I think to myself, our life feels pretty much like the Old Normal—and it's really a wonderful life.

TIPS ➢ ➢ ➢

1. Don't grow impatient if your wife still seems tired. The number one post-treatment side effect is fatigue—from shock, stress, fear, depression, and sleep deprivation because of hot flashes.
2. You can still be your wife's appointment pal. Tag along for her periodic round of cancer checkups. She'll likely be grateful for the company.
3. You and your wife both may feel motivated to change for the better—eating healthier, exercising more. But don't overdo it, or the changes likely won't stick. "I encourage people to make changes based on what makes sense to them, what fits their lifestyle, what gives them more energy," says psychologist Morry Edwards Ph.D., a Michigan psychologist who works with cancer patients and is the author of *MindBody Cancer Wellness: A Self-Help Stress Management Manual.*

➢ BONUS TIP

The amount of breast cancer information is supposed to double in the next 5 years. To find out about new therapies that could benefit your wife (and, by extension, you and your family), sign up for free e-mail updates at www.breastcancer.org.

Glossary

A cancer patient and her spouse need to keep abreast, if I may use that word, of the unfamiliar words and phrases that assault them during diagnosis and treatment.

I've tried to include the terms that you're most likely to hear and that will give you a clearer sense of your wife's condition. This glossary is adapted from a thorough booklet called *Breast Cancer Dictionary*, available from the American Cancer Society (800-227-2345 or www.cancer.org) and from the incredibly helpful *Talking Dictionary* at www.breastcancer.org, in which celebrities and doctors speak the terms and definitions aloud, so you'll always remember that "in situ" is pronounced "in SYE-too," (rhymes with "why" as in, "why me?") and not "in SIH-too." Your fine pronunciation won't get you better care, but it may make you feel a little less uncertain as you tread the unfamiliar terrain of cancer world.

absolute survival benefit: The benefit that a treatment such as chemotherapy has for a patient. Absolute survival benefit is given as a percentile—the number of women in a group of 100 whose cancer won't recur because of chemo.

adjuvant therapy: Adjuvant simply means "helpful" or "additional." This somewhat intimidating phrase refers to treatments besides the main treatment for cancer, which is the surgical removal of the tumor. Adjuvant therapy includes chemotherapy, radiation, and hormone therapy (various anticancer pills).

alopecia: Baldness. That's what many chemo cocktails cause. To apply for wig reimbursement, your wife will need a prescription for the wig. This is one of the terms that will appear on the prescription.

alternative therapy: An unproven treatment chosen instead of standard therapy.

antiemetic: An antinausea or antivomiting drug. Antiemetics are given before chemo, and your wife will keep a stock at home as well.

axilla: Armpit area.

axillary dissection: Taking out lymph nodes in the armpit (to check for cancer).

benign: No evidence of cancer.

bilateral: On both sides of the body. Bilateral breast cancer means a tumor in each breast.

biopsy: Removing a sample of tissue to see if cancer cells are present. The standard of care for breast biopsies is to remove a core of tissue with a needle rather than to remove the lump surgically.

breast conservation: Preserving the breast by removing only the cancer and a small area of benign tissue surrounding the tumor.

breast prosthesis: A silicone- or fiber-filled object worn in a bra to replace a breast that was surgically removed.

calcifications: Small calcium deposits in the breast, typically discovered by mammography. Benign breast disease can cause calcifications; so can cancer. A biopsy may be required.

cancer cell: A cell that divides and reproduces abnormally and has the potential to spread throughout the body, crowding out normal cells and tissue.

chemotherapy: Treatment with drugs to destroy cancer cells or to make them less active.

clear margins: "Margins" of tissue around the tumor that are free of cancer. In a lumpectomy, the surgeon removes margins of tissue that surround the tumor in all directions. If there's no cancer, the margins are clear and there's no need for further surgery to treat that particular cancer. If the margins aren't clear, the doctor may feel that another surgery will remove the remaining cancer—or that a mastectomy is recommended.

clinical trials: These trials test how well new medical treatments or other medical practices work in people. Each study is designed to test screening, prevention, diagnosis, or treatment of disease. For information on breast cancer trials, contact the National Cancer Institute at (800) 422-6237 or www.cancer.gov/clinical_trials/.

complementary therapy: Therapies used along with standard therapy, including acupuncture, herbal supplements, and more. Before trying any such therapy, even vitamins, a patient should ask her doctor if there is the possibility of a negative interaction with her standard treatment.

cranial prosthesis: No, not a new head—a wig. That's the term that will go on the doctor's prescription that enables your wife to file for medical reimbursement for her hair hat.

differentiation: How the cells in a breast tumor stack up to normal breast cells in terms of maturity. Well-differentiated breast cancer cells resemble regular breast cells; they're also slow growers. Poorly differentiated or undifferentiated cancer cells don't look or act like regular cells. They're rapid growers, and they tend to spread throughout the body. (See "grade.")

duct: In a breast, the passage through which milk travels from the milk-making lobule to the nipple.

epoetin (brand names: Epogen, Procrit, Eprex): A drug that helps the body make more red blood cells. It is administered to chemotherapy patients whose red blood count is low.

estrogen: The female sex hormone produced mainly by the ovaries.

estrogen receptor assay: A lab test of the breast cancer to see if it has estrogen receptors—that is, if estrogen will stimulate the cancer's growth. ER-positive cancers usually respond well to hormonal therapies; ER-negative cancers usually don't.

grade: An assessment of the cancer's degree of abnormality, ranging from I to III. As in golf, a low score is better. The higher the grade, the greater the degree of abnormality and the greater the risk of the cancer's rapid growth and spread.

HER2/neu gene: A gene responsible for production of the HER2/neu protein. This protein is present in small amounts on the outer surface of normal breast cells. About a quarter to a third of breast cancers have an abnormal HER2/neu gene that causes an excess of the protein to be produced, which tends to result in a more aggressive cancer. This type of cancer can be treated with a targeted therapy called Herceptin.

hormonal therapy: Cancer treatment that removes, blocks, or adds hormones.

in situ: Cancer confined to its point of origin—the breast ducts in the case of breast cancer.

invasive breast cancer: Cancer that has spread from the milk glands (lobules) or milk passages (ducts) where it began to nearby fatty breast tissue. Also called infiltrating cancer.

lesion: An area of abnormal tissue change—and a less emotionally charged synonym for tumor.

lobules: The glands in a woman's breast that produce milk.

lump: A mass in the breast or elsewhere in the body.

lumpectomy: Surgery to remove the tumor in the breast and a small amount of normal tissue around it (just to make sure the tumor has been completely cut out).

lymph node: Bean-shaped (and -sized) collections of immune system tissue that filter cell waste from lymphatic fluid. Also known as lymph glands.

lymphatic system: Tissues and organs that produce, store, and carry the body's infection-fighting white blood cells. Invasive breast cancer sometimes penetrates lymphatic channels and spreads to lymph nodes.

lymphedema: Swelling caused by excess fluid in the arms or legs. The removal of lymph nodes and radiation can put a breast cancer patient at lifelong risk of lymphedema in the arm on the side of the affected breast.

malignant: Cancerous.

marker: An indicator from a blood test of possible cancer activity in the body. The tests for "markers" may help in diagnosing metastatic disease, but they have limitations. A normal level does not prove a patient is cancer-free; a high level does not always mean the cancer has recurred or progressed. While they may help along the road to diagnosis of metastatic disease, cancer markers have not yet translated into better survival for women with breast cancer.

mastectomy: Surgical removal of the breast.

medical oncologist: A doctor who is trained to diagnose and treat cancer with chemotherapy and other drugs. In patient lingo, this doc is usually referred to as the oncologist.

metastasis: The spread of cancer cells from the breast to other parts of the body via the lymph system or the bloodstream.

needle biopsy: Removal of fluid, cells, or tissue with a needle for examination under a microscope to check for cancer.

negative: There's no cancer found in the tumor, lymph nodes, or organs tested.

neoadjuvant therapy: Treatment given before the main treatment (which would be surgery in the case of breast cancer) to create more favorable conditions for the surgery. Chemotherapy, for example, is sometimes given before surgery to shrink the tumor, making it easier to remove and sometimes making a lumpectomy possible, instead of a mastectomy.

Neupogen: If chemotherapy wipes out too many white blood cells, this drug can be injected to stimulate the bone marrow to make more of them.

no evidence of disease: Exactly what it says. But keep in mind that NED, as doctors call this condition, is not the same as free of disease. Undetected cancer cells may still lurk.

oncologist: A doctor trained to diagnose and treat cancer. Your wife will be treated by several kinds of oncologists: surgical, medical, and radiation.

pathologist: A doctor who determines if the tumor is benign or cancerous, and who assigns a grade to the cancer.

port [also called a port-a-cath]: A small device placed under the skin. It empties into a blood vessel and makes it easier to give chemotherapy and to take blood for tests.

positive: Yes, there is cancer in the tumor or lymph node or organ in question.

primary site: The place where the cancer begins.

prophylactic mastectomy: Removing one or both breasts to reduce the risk of developing breast cancer.

radiation oncologist: A doctor who treats the patient with radiation to wipe out any lingering cancer cells and prevent a recurrence in the breast.

radiation therapy: Bombarding the breast (and possibly the armpit as well) with x-rays to damage and destroy any cancer cells that remain after surgery.

radiologist: A doctor who reads mammograms and can perform breast biopsies using a needle.

reconstruction: Building a new breast with implants or tissue from the patient's body after a mastectomy.

recurrence: Cancer that comes back, either in the breast (a local recurrence), in nearby lymph nodes (regional recurrence), or in organs such as the lungs, liver, bones, or brain (distant recurrence).

regional involvement: Cancer that has spread to nearby areas like the lymph nodes of the armpit, but not to organs or to the bones.

remission: A decrease in or disappearance of signs and symptoms of cancer. Partial remission means some, but not all, signs and symptoms have disappeared.

Complete remission means all signs and symptoms of cancer have disappeared, although cancer cells may still be present in the body.

sentinel node biopsy: Guided by blue dye or a radioactive tracer, the surgeon removes the first node or nodes that breast cancer would probably reach in the armpit area. At some hospitals, the pathologist checks the sentinel node or nodes for cancer while the lumpectomy or mastectomy is going on. (At other hospitals, the patient must wait 5 to 7 days for results.) Word comes back to the operating room: cancer (which means more nodes will be removed to see the extent of the spread) or no cancer (which means no additional nodes will be removed).

staging: Where your wife stands on the cancer spectrum. The range is from Stage 0 to Stage IV, based on tumor size, lymph node involvement, and the nature of her cancer. Stages 0 to II are "early." Stage III is locally advanced, and Stage IV is advanced with spread to other organs. (See page 118 for more information on staging.)

surgical biopsy: The doctor cuts into the breast and takes a sample of the lesion to determine if it is cancerous or not. Also known as excisional biopsy.

surgical oncologist: A surgeon who specializes in cutting out cancer.

survival rate: The number of people who survive a certain period of time after diagnosis (the typical time period used in survival rates is 5 years). If your wife's survival rate is 85 percent, then after 5 years, 85 out of 100 breast cancer patients with a similar prognosis are alive and well.

systemic disease: Breast cancer that affects the whole body.

systemic treatment: Therapies that affect cells throughout the body. For example, chemotherapy is systemic, while surgery and radiation are targeted to the site of the cancer.

tamoxifen: The most common hormonal therapy, administered for 5 years to patients who might benefit. Tamoxifen blocks the ability of estrogen to reach a cancer cell that would be stimulated to grow from the estrogen.

tumor: An abnormal lump or mass of tissue; it can be cancerous or not cancerous.

vaginal lubricant: An over-the-counter remedy for the vaginal dryness that can be a side effect of chemo drugs, the premature push into menopause caused by chemo, or hormonal therapies like tamoxifen.

white blood cells: Cells that help fight infection and disease. Chemotherapy can reduce the number of white blood cells.

Experts

Many doctors, nurses, therapists, and social workers were instrumental in shaping this book.

Susan Abrams, a Maryland oncological social worker

Katherine Alley, M.D., a breast surgeon and medical director of the Suburban Breast Center in Bethesda, Maryland

Cecelia Brennecke, M.D., director of breast imaging at the John Hopkins Breast Center at Greenspring Station in Baltimore

Adam Brufsky, M.D., codirector of the Magee-Womens Breast Cancer Program in Pittsburgh

Patricia Clark, a nurse practitioner at the University of Michigan, Ann Arbor, and an oncology nurse

Anne Coscarelli, Ph.D., director of the UCLA Ted Mann Family Resource Center at the Jonsson Comprehensive Cancer Center in Los Angeles

Cynthia Drogula, M.D., a breast surgeon in Washington, D.C.

Morry Edwards, Ph.D., a Michigan psychologist and author of *MindBody Cancer Wellness: A Self-Help Stress Management Manual*

Irene Gage, M.D., a radiation oncologist who practices at Sibley Memorial Hospital in Washington, D.C.

Patricia Ganz, M.D., an oncologist who is a professor of health services and medicine at the UCLA Schools of Medicine and Public Health

Sharon Giordano, M.D., an assistant professor in the department of breast oncology at the University of Texas M.D. Anderson Cancer Center in Houston

William Goodson, M.D., a breast surgeon and senior clinical research scientist at the California Pacific Medical Center Research Institute in San Francisco

Carolyn Hendricks, M.D., an oncologist who practices in Montgomery County, Maryland, and primarily treats breast cancer patients

Claudine Isaacs, M.D., an oncologist at Georgetown University's Lombardi Cancer Center in Washington, D.C.

Ronnie Kaye, a therapist, breast cancer survivor, and author of *Spinning Straw into Gold: Your Emotional Recovery from Breast Cancer*

Roz Kleban, administrative supervisor of social work services at the Memorial Sloan-Kettering Cancer Center in New York City

Matthew Loscalzo, director of patient and family support services at the University of California at San Diego Cancer Center

Jean Lynn, an oncology nurse who is the program director for the Breast Care Center at George Washington University Medical Faculty Associates in Washington, D.C.

Mary Ann McCabe, Ph.D., a licensed clinical psychologist and associate professor at the George Washington University School of Medicine in Washington, D.C.

Frank McCaffrey, a social worker who counsels breast cancer husbands at Boston's Beth Israel Deaconess Medical Center

Kathleen McCue, a child life specialist, social worker, and director of children's programs at The Gathering Place in Beachwood, Ohio

Sharon Manne, Ph.D., a psychologist and director of the psycho-oncology program at the Fox Chase Cancer Center in Philadelphia

Venus Masselam, Ph.D., a psychologist in Bethesda, Maryland

Mary Jane Massie, M.D., a psychiatrist at Memorial Sloan-Kettering Cancer Center in New York City

Beth Meyerowitz, Ph.D., a professor of psychology and preventive medicine at the University of Southern California

Megan Mills, Ph.D., director of psychosocial oncology at Chicago's Rush Cancer Institute

Maurice Nahabedian, M.D., director of the plastic surgery group at the Johns Hopkins Breast Center in Baltimore

Anne Nickodem, M.D., a plastic surgeon who practices in Virginia and Maryland

Sherwin Nuland, M.D., Yale University clinical professor of surgery and author of *How We Live* and *How We Die*

Anne O'Connor, a care coordinator nurse at Georgetown University's Lombardi Cancer Center in Washington, D.C.

Richard Ogden, Ph.D., a Bethesda, Maryland, psychologist who runs a support group for breast cancer husbands

Michael Olding, M.D., associate professor of surgery and chief of the Division of Plastic and Reconstructive Surgery at George Washington University in Washington, D.C.

Julia Rowland, Ph.D., who runs the Office of Cancer Survivorship at the National Cancer Institute in Bethesda, Maryland

Hester Hill Schnipper, chief of oncology social work at Boston's Beth Israel Deaconess Medical Center and author of *After Breast Cancer: A Common-Sense Guide to Life After Treatment*

Leslie Schover, Ph.D., a professor of behavioral science in the cancer prevention division at the University of Texas M.D. Anderson Cancer Center in Houston

Mikkael Sekeres, M.D., co-editor of *Facing Cancer* and an assistant professor in the hematology-oncology department at the Cleveland Clinic Lerner College of Medicine

Cleveland Shields, Ph.D., a marriage and family therapist and an associate professor at the University of Rochester

Lillie Shockney, a nurse, breast cancer survivor, and director of education and outreach at the Johns Hopkins Breast Center in Baltimore

Robert Siegel, M.D., director of hematology and oncology at George Washington University Medical Faculty Associates in Washington, D.C.

Frederick P. Smith, M.D., a medical oncologist who practices in Chevy Chase, Maryland

Janet Sobel, a physical therapist who practices in the Washington, D.C., area and works with breast cancer patients, specializing in lymphedema

Patricia Spicer, an oncology social worker and coordinator of the breast cancer program for the national organization CancerCare

David Spiegel, associate chair of psychiatry at the Stanford University School of Medicine

Annette Stanton, Ph.D., a health psychologist and professor in the UCLA department of psychology

Jill Taylor-Brown, director of psychosocial oncology and supportive care at CancerCare Manitoba

Kyle Terrell, a surgical oncology nurse practitioner at the Johns Hopkins Breast Center in Baltimore

Theodore Tsangaris, M.D., medical director of the Johns Hopkins Breast Center in Baltimore

Victor Vogel, M.D., an oncologist and director of the Magee/University of Pittsburgh Cancer Institute Breast Cancer Prevention Program

Karen Weihs, M.D., a professor of psychiatry and behavioral sciences at George Washington University in Washington, D.C.

Marisa Weiss, M.D., a Philadelphia breast radiation oncologist and founder and president of the nonprofit organization and Web site breastcancer.org

Tzipi Weiss, Ph.D., visiting assistant professor at Long Island University, C. W. Post campus

Jim Zabora, Sc.D., dean of the School of Social Service at the Catholic University of America in Washington, D.C.

Index

Boldface page references indicate illustrations. Underscored references indicate boxed text.

C

D

E

F

G

H

I

J

K

L

M

N

O

P

R

S

T

V

W